I0487611

THE NECK STEP

BY
DR. DONNIE LABORDE

ILLUSTRATED BY
ALLYSON LABORDE

Bloomington, IN 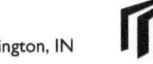 Milton Keynes, UK

authorHOUSE™

AuthorHouse™
1663 Liberty Drive, Suite 200
Bloomington, IN 47403
www.authorhouse.com
Phone: 1-800-839-8640

AuthorHouse™ UK Ltd.
500 Avebury Boulevard
Central Milton Keynes, MK9 2BE
www.authorhouse.co.uk
Phone: 08001974150

© 2006 Dr. Donnie Laborde. All rights reserved.

No part of this book may be reproduced, stored in a retrieval system, or transmitted by any means without the written permission of the author.

First published by AuthorHouse 10/5/2006

ISBN: 1-4259-3572-9 (sc)

Printed in the United States of America
Bloomington, Indiana

This book is printed on acid-free paper.

DEDICATION

Are you one of the many people suffering from symptoms such as headaches, dizziness, neck pain, ringing in the ears, loss of coordination, blurred vision, memory loss, unusual sensations, or pain in the arms? Has no one, including your doctor, taken your complaints seriously? Then this book was written for you.

The information in this section is vital to starting you on the path to understanding your symptoms. The average sufferer is run through a typical routine: numerous tests, various treatments, and visits to several different doctors. This routine generally results in the sufferer concluding they will just have to live with the symptoms and pain.

Patients usually continue taking medications, receiving only temporary relief. In some cases, patients start to believe their problems exist only in their mind, with some doctors actually referring patients to pain management care with psychological counseling.

If these paragraphs describe what you
have been living through, then take *The Neck Step*.

It is very likely that at some point in your life, prior to the onset of symptoms, you experienced an injury to your neck. It might have been so subtle or may have occurred so long ago you cannot even recall the incident. Perhaps it was a slight fender-bender in a parking lot with no immediate pain or obvious symptoms.

Then, without warning, maybe years later, the signs started. Your body began to let you know that something wasn't right. The doctor who examined you probably never considered what might be the main cause: the dorsal primary nerve. This will be discussed in detail in chapter 3.

Your treatment only targeted your symptoms and not the cause. In this case, you can only experience short-term relief, if any, and you continue to suffer.

The Neck Step was written so that you can finally learn the causes of your symptoms and seek treatment accordingly.

INTRODUCTION

Are you completely and absolutely fed up with your symptoms? Are you tired of living with your problem, or taking pain medication only to temporarily relieve your symptoms, then having your aggravating problem only return later? Are you ready to understand your possible and probable problem causing your symptoms? Then you need to take *The Neck Step*!

We have seven neck bones in our neck. Muscles move these bones around our inner spinal cord. Rubber bands called ligaments hold our bones together. Sensory nerves in the joints of our neck bones, and in these ligaments, monitor the neck bones movement. If you damage these rubber bands (ligaments) allowing the neck bones to move abnormally, then these sensory nerves in our neck get irritated. This leads to symptoms of neck pain, headaches, dizziness, blurred vision, loss of balance, etc. You should take *The Neck Step* to understand more.

Table of Contents

CHAPTER I

UNDERSTAND YOUR PROBLEM

The world that we have created is a result of the level of thinking we have done in the past, solutions exist at a higher level of thinking.

– Albert Einstein

Taking *The Neck Step* will lead you toward discovering a solution to your symptoms. This book is based on a Biblical principle found in Proverbs 4:7, which says, "Wisdom is the principle thing, therefore get wisdom and in all thy getting, get understanding."

Understanding is the first step to determining a solution. We must first understand the cause of the problem. Symptoms that continue to return are an indication you are probably not receiving treatment aimed at removing the cause. It is likely no one has ever explained this cause to you, and just as likely they are not sure just what that cause is.

The Neck Step aims not just to reveal possible causes for your symptoms, but also to help you understand the steps you should take to begin a true healing process. The knowledge you gain from this book will help you participate in your diagnosis and play an active role in treatment.

Understanding the causes of your problem will allow you to take control of the healing process, and help you to know what activities you do that might aggravate your symptoms and slow the healing process.

Proverbs 4:7 can apply to understanding your body, but also to your life. Wisdom is important, but understanding is vital! Everyone has the capacity for knowledge, but we must be given the opportunity to understand.

Chapter II

Your Neck/Normal Anatomy

Your neck is very simply complicated. In order to understand the dynamics of your neck, we must first take a look at the anatomical structure.

The neck has seven bones (vertebrae), separated by a cushion of fibro cartilage, called an intervertebral disc. [Figure 1] There is not a disc between the first and second neck (cervical) bones. The disc resembles a sunny side up egg when looking from above down. [Figure 2]

The nucleus in the center of the disc is very unique. It has the ability to absorb water, especially at night when you are laying down putting no axial pressure, (the pressure from the weight of your head and body straight down on your spine standing or sitting), on your disc. You are actually slightly taller in the morning due to this nucleus absorption. As the day wears on your disc with pressure from above – down, the nucleus will lose this water retention and you will be slightly shorter. As we get older, the disc loses this ability to grow in height, and this is one reason why we are not as tall as we used to be. This is also why astronauts grow taller in space (lack of gravity), yet lose their gained height once they have been back on earth for a short time.

The nucleus is slightly anterior in relation to the vertebrae and the disc is also thicker in the front. This will cause the neck to form a c-shaped curve in the neck and act like a shock absorber, as we walk, bounce, jump, etc. in life. The disc, due to its thickness, allows flexibility of your neck.

In the center of your cervical vertebra is a canal where your spinal cord runs. [Figure 3] Your brain communicates with your body through this cord. The information from your body, like pain, pressure, etc., runs through this cord to your brain, and your brain's response or control of your body runs back down this cord, back out to your body. If this cord was damaged, as in a neck bone fracture, putting pressure on the cord, your brain could not control your body below this damaged area. There are also holes (canals) in the sides of your neck. [Figure 4] These allow the nerve to exit your neck from the spinal cord and control your neck and arms. These nerves (spinal nerves) will be discussed later in detail.

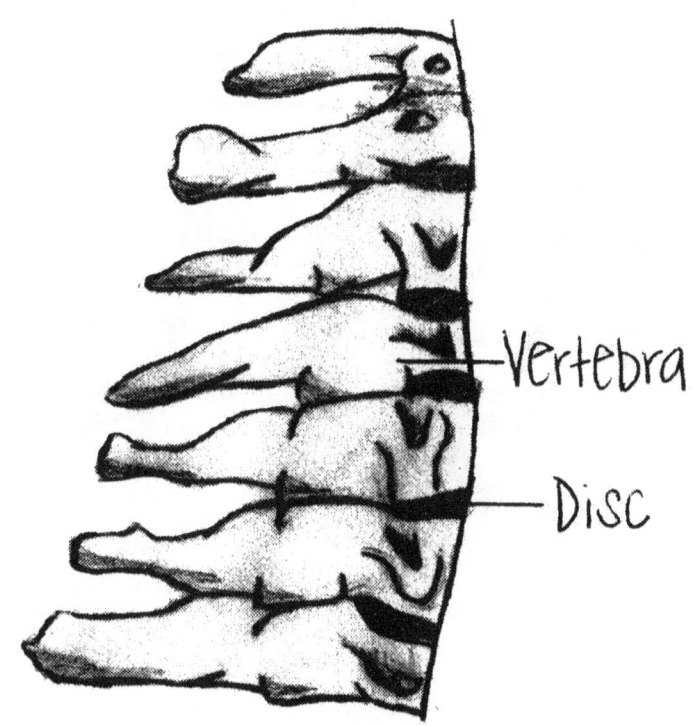

FIGURE 1

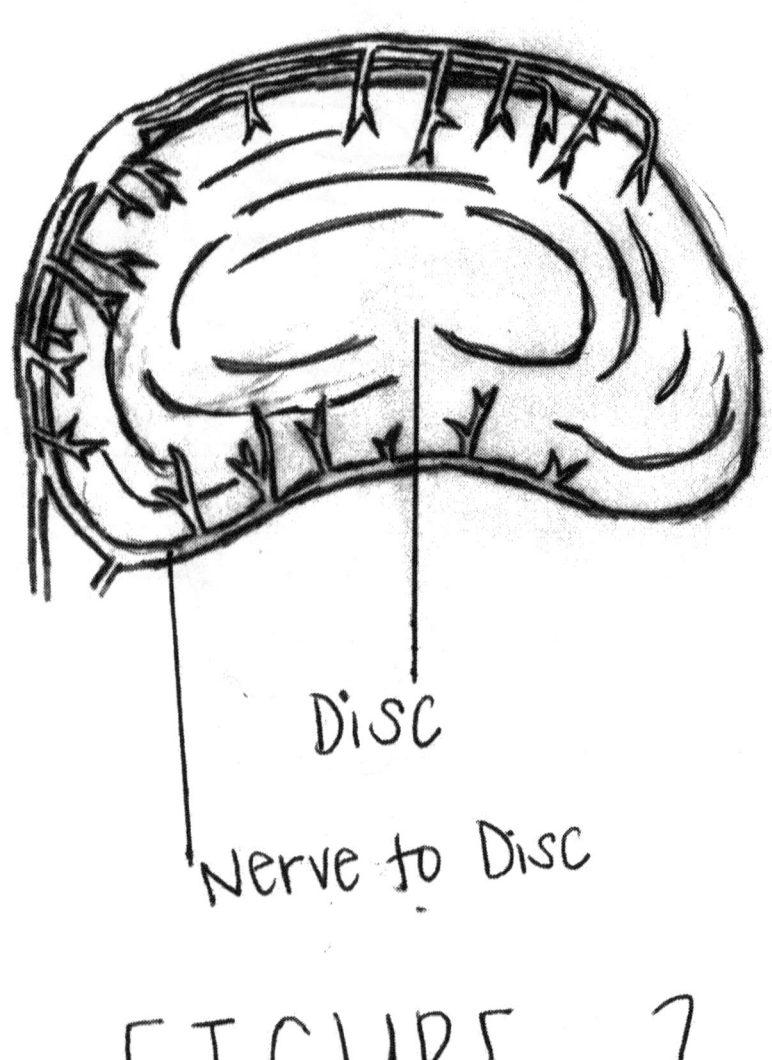

Disc

Nerve to Disc

FIGURE 2

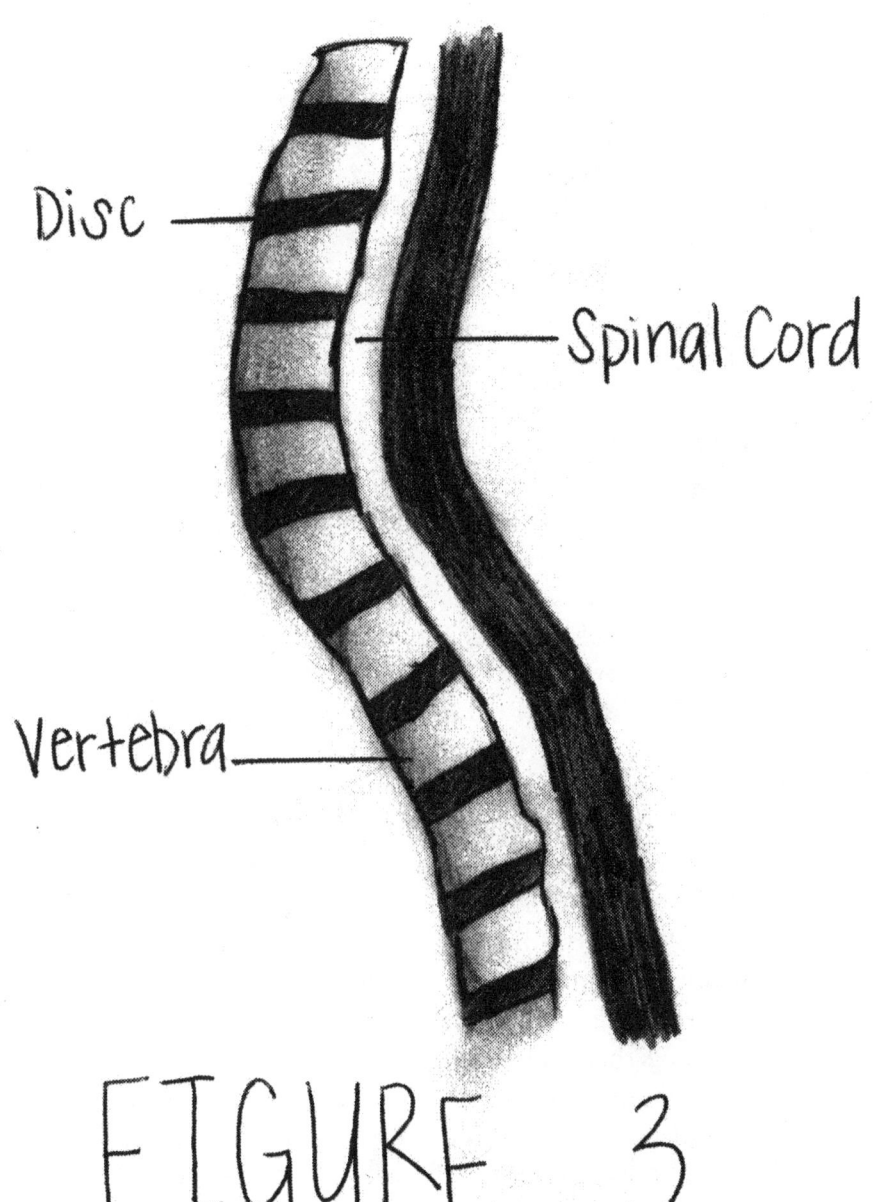

Disc

Spinal Cord

Vertebra

FIGURE 3

The muscles surrounding your neck move your head in all directions. The design of your neck bones, together with the disc, allows your neck to be quite flexible. During this movement, however, it is vital the bones do not hit the spinal cord and the spinal nerves. It is imperative the bones in the neck move dynamically smooth. Any alteration of the movement of the neck bones can irritate or damage these nerves causing symptoms of pain, headaches, dizziness, etc.

This is why the bones are surrounded by tough, but flexible fibrous connective tissue called ligaments. [Figure 5] I like to call these ligaments tough rubber bands. In reality, that is exactly what they act like. They will stretch when you move your neck, but will spring back to original form when you move your head back. In order to understand your possible need for treatment of your damaged neck, you first must know a few basic facts about these ligaments.

Ligaments are bands of fibrous tissue connecting bones, allowing for movement between these bones. Ligaments are formed from cells called fibroblasts. These fibroblasts secrete fibers to form and strengthen the ligaments. A key point to make here is that fibroblasts lay down fibers to strengthen a ligament. The directions these fibers are laid down are the specific direction of the stress applied to this ligament. For instance, if a ligament between two bones is constantly stretched forward, the fibroblast will lay down more fibers to increase the strength when the movement remains forward. If the bones are stressed sideways all of a sudden for the first time, this ligament will not be ready for the task, due to not having been previously stressed in that direction to allow the fibroblast to lay down the needed fibers. This is the same principal that tells how the fibroblasts function to restore a damaged ligament back to its near original strength (discussed later).

Ligaments are mainly collagen fibers. Collagen, when mature becomes three procollagen chains intertwining together with cross-links holding them together. [Figure 6] This collagen triple-helix structure gives the ligament its strength. The flexibility of a ligament comes from a substance called elastin, which is mixed in with the collagen within a ligament. Elastin has the ability to be flexible and elastic like.

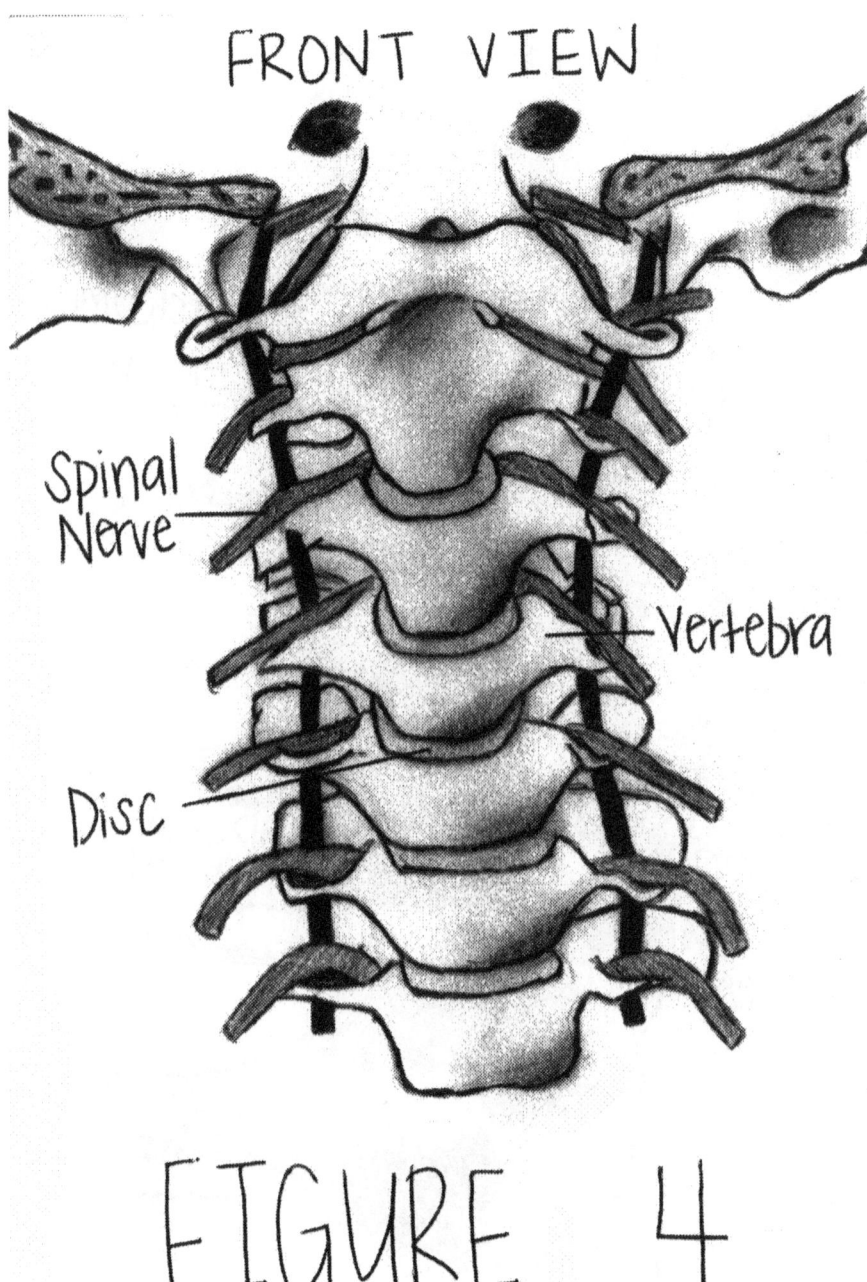

FRONT VIEW

Spinal Nerve

Vertebra

Disc

FIGURE 4

FIGURE 5

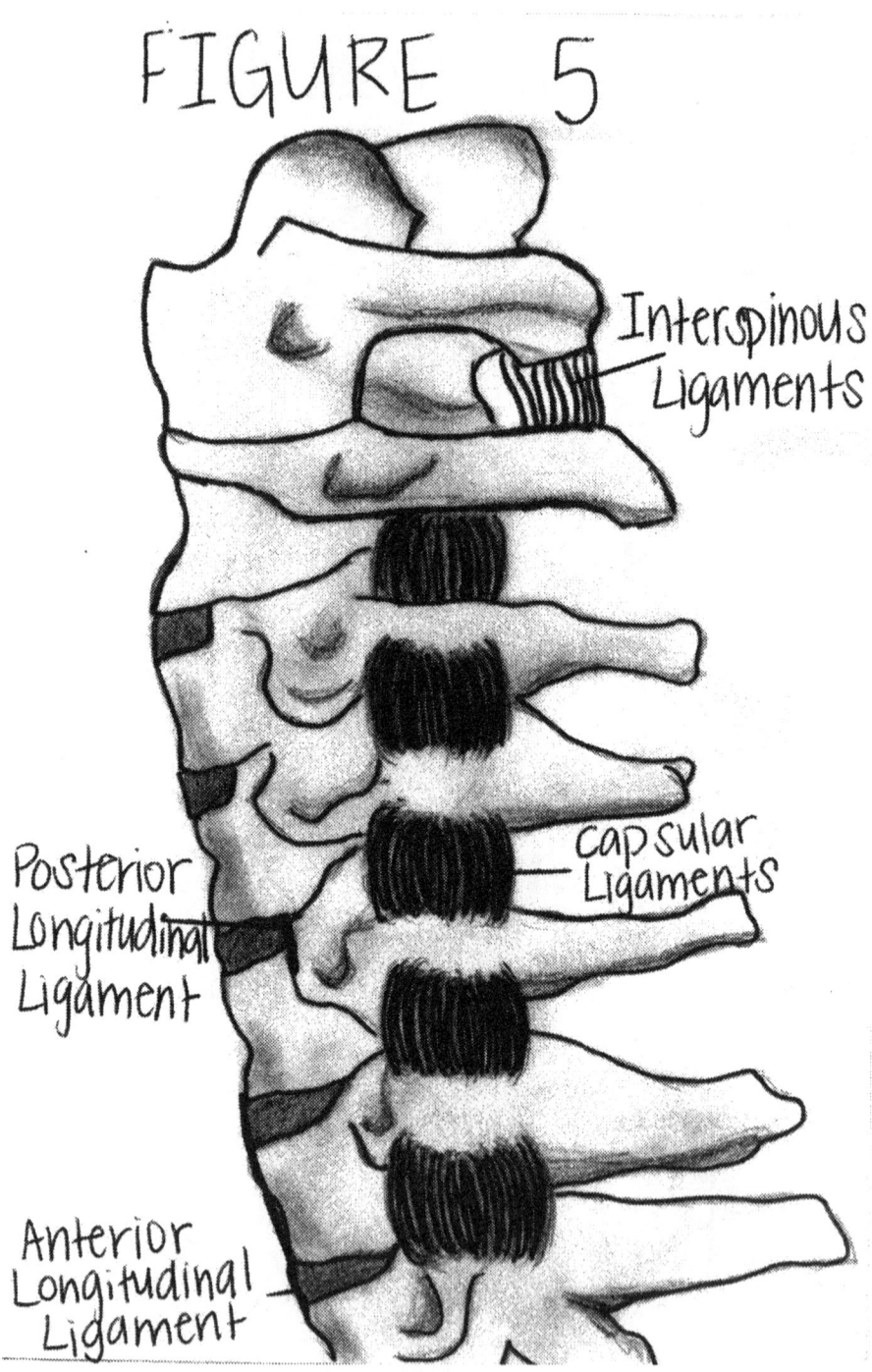

Interspinous
Ligaments

Capsular
Ligaments

Posterior
Longitudinal
Ligament

Anterior
Longitudinal
Ligament

Part of the blood supply to the brain goes through each side of the neck bones. This blood vessel is called the vertebral artery, which goes through holes called the vertebral foramen. [Figure 7] Obviously altered motion could damage this vessel.

SUMMARY:

Your neck bones move in all directions, giving your head the mobility necessary for everyday living. Muscles, which surround your neck, move your neck bones around vital spinal nerves going to your neck and arms, spinal cord going down your spine, and vertebral arteries, supplying your brain with blood. Tough rubber bands, called ligaments hold these bones together, allowing movement in all directions without hitting or damaging these nerves or blood vessels. The direction of stress applied to these ligaments will signal the fibroblast to lay down new fibers in these lines of stress, to strengthen the ligament.

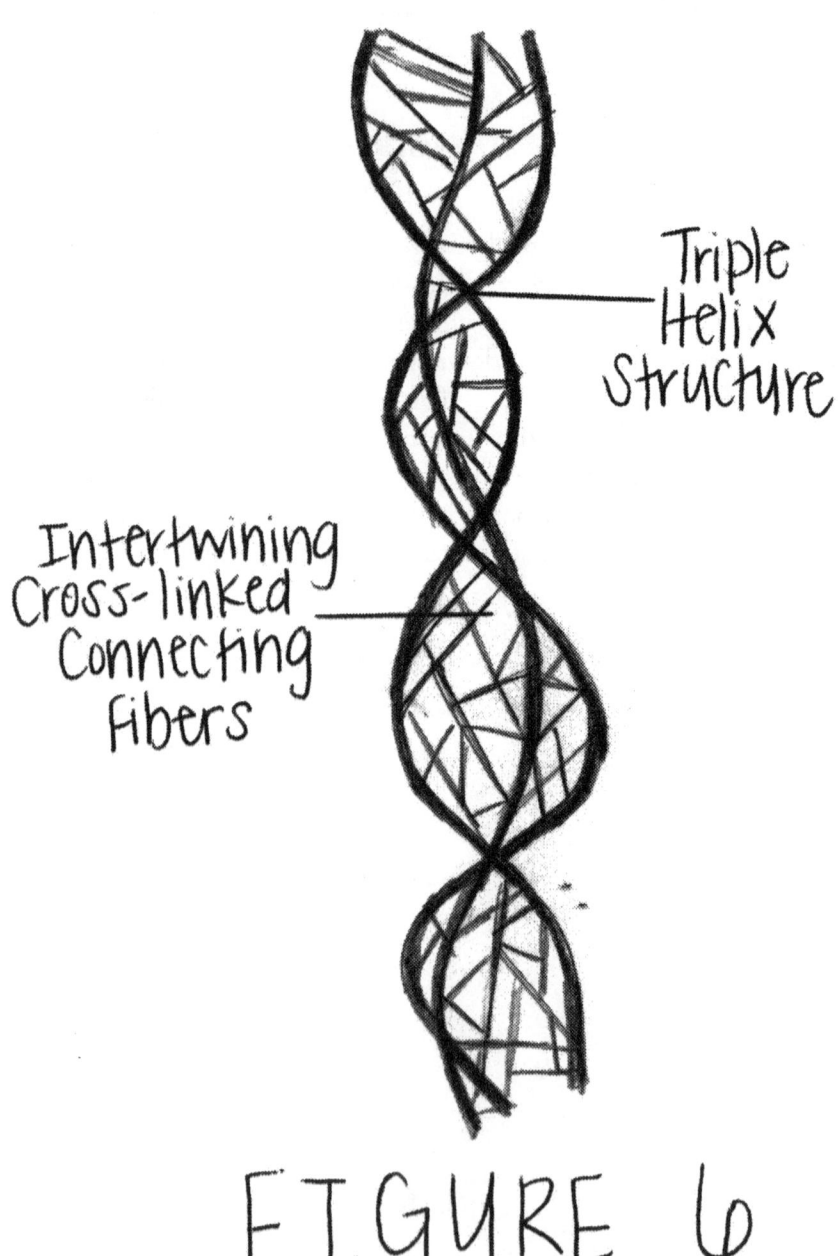

Triple
Helix
Structure

Intertwining
Cross-linked
Connecting
Fibers

FIGURE 6

FIGURE 7

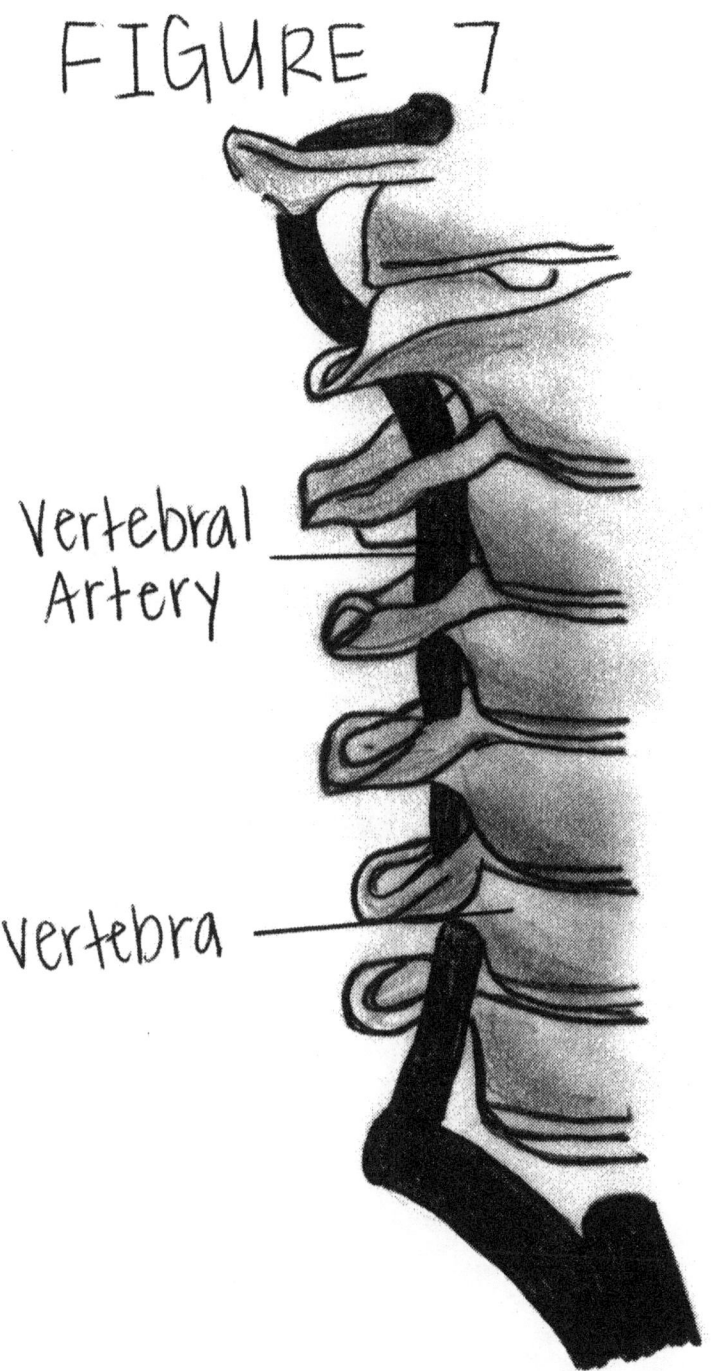

Vertebral Artery

Vertebra

CHAPTER III

THE NERVE

In this chapter we are going to begin explaining how a specific nerve in your neck may be causing your symptoms. Before we start getting into abnormal nerve functions, we need to first understand normal nerve function.

In order to stay alive, the nerves in the body aid in controlling its needs. This is known as homeostasis. For instance, there are specific nerve receptors checking for the proper amount of oxygen in your blood. If the oxygen content is low, these nerves will let the nervous system know and cause motor nerves to react. In this case the reaction is to start breathing deeper, move often, and increase your heart rate to pump more blood. This requires the nerves to have two base parts. These parts include sensory and motor. Sensory detects problems and motor reacts and solves the problems.

The nerves coming from your spine to your body have both sensory and motor fibers in them, including the specific nerve that may be causing your symptoms. The following discussion is specifically about the nerves in your neck.

Your brain controls your arms through spinal nerves exiting your neck. There are seven cervical (neck) vertebrae. These are known as C1 through C7. The C stands for cervical. There are eight cervical spinal nerves known as C1 through C8. [Figure 8]

As the spinal nerve exits the vertebra, the nerve splits into two separate nerves. [Figure 9] The nerve in the front, the Ventral Ramus, runs into the arms. The Ventral Ramus is responsible for sensory (pain, touch, pressure, etc.) and motor control (muscle contraction) of the arms.

If you go to a doctor because of pain in your arms, the doctor will check this Ventral Ramus several different ways. For instance, to check the Ventral Ramus of C5, the sensory would be tested by running a pinwheel (needle-like apparatus) down the biceps. The C5 motor would be tested by muscle testing the biceps and checking its deep tendon reflex with a reflex hammer. The Ventral Ramus nerves can be objectively tested by other ways such as an EMG, which is an electric current sent through a Ventral Ramus nerve to test its conductivity.

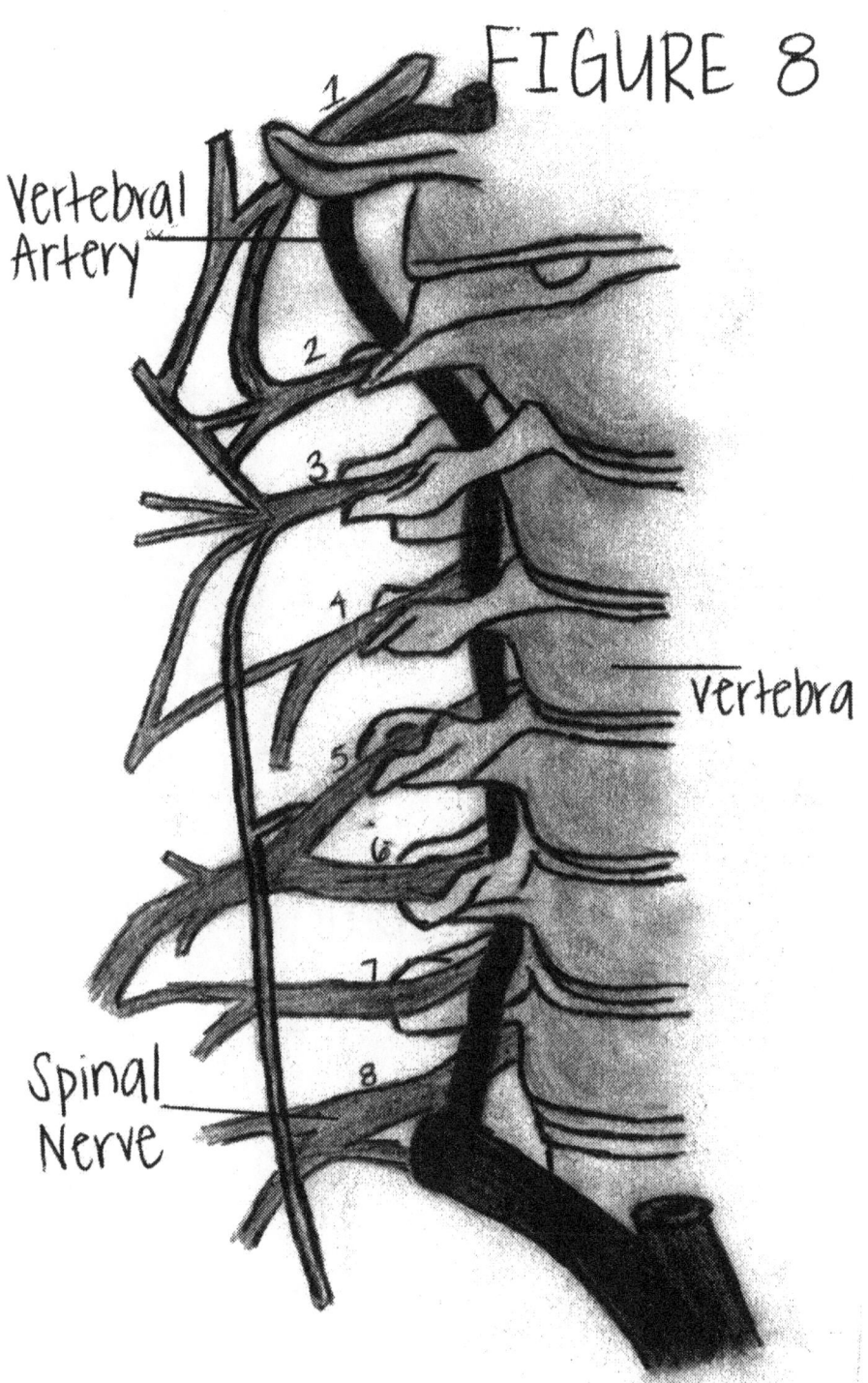

FIGURE 8

Vertebral Artery

Vertebra

Spinal Nerve

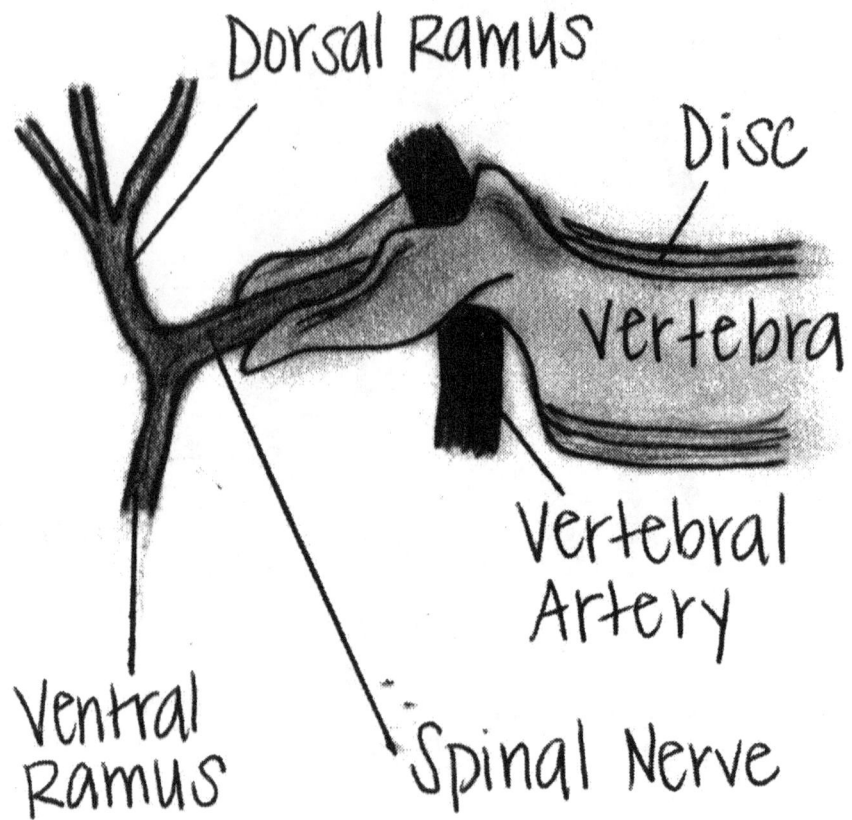

FIGURE 9

If you have been to a doctor for your symptoms, the doctor has probably tested the Ventral Ramus, which is the anterior half of the spinal nerve. This book is not about this Ventral Ramus. It is about the posterior half, the Dorsal Ramus (The Nerve). The Dorsal Ramus does not go down the arms. As it exits the cervical vertebra, it branches into three different nerves, [Figure 9]: the medial, communicating, and lateral branch. These branches supply the neck muscles and joints. These nerves supply sensory and motor (muscle) to your neck.

The Dorsal Ramus may be the key source of your symptoms, which to date probably has not even been considered. To understand this, we need to look deeper into the medial branch of the Dorsal Ramus. The Dorsal Ramus is "The Nerve" monitoring and protecting against any altered movement of the cervical vertebra that could possibly harm the spinal cord, spinal nerves, or vertebral artery. The Dorsal Ramus accomplishes the monitoring of the cervical vertebra by supplying sensory nerves that are in the joints of the neck, as well as in the ligaments and tendons of the neck. These sensory nerves are known as mechanoreceptors.

These mechanoreceptors in the neck could be the source of your symptoms. Keep in mind these mechanoreceptors are only a monitoring device letting the brain know if the cervical vertebra is not moving correctly. Therefore, the actual source of your problem is probably coming from altered motion, not a defect or malfunction of these sensory nerves.

The following explanation of the mechanoreceptors received input from tapes of a lecture from Dr. Barry Wyke, Director of the Neurological Unit of the Royal College of Surgeons in England.

Remember nerves sense pain as well as sense movement. Mechanoreceptors are placed in strategic areas of the neck for communication to the brain. There are three different types of mechanoreceptors, which communicate with several different locations in the brain to let the brain know what movement is taking place, where the movement is, and especially if the movement is too much that is taking place and coordinates the muscles to allow for smooth movement. The fewer mechanoreceptors in a joint, the less coordinated the movement will be. Did you catch that point? I guess that means Michael Jordan has a zillion more mechanoreceptors than I do.

The vertebrae in the neck have joints in the back, known as facet joints. [Figure 10] These joints move over each other when you move your neck. Therefore, they need continuous lubrication. To keep this lubrication fluid in these joints, a capsule with synovial tissue surrounds them. This synovial tissue is located in joints throughout the body called synovial joints, as in the facet joints of the cervical spine. All synovial joints of the body, without exception, are provided with mechanoreceptors. When these joints move, the mechanoreceptors let the brain know where and how much they move. They aid in fine purposeful skilled movement.

As we get older, or if these mechanoreceptors are damaged by trauma, arthritis, or immobility of the joint, this will cause a loss of these receptors and therefore a loss of fine and gross motor skills. You will not be stable walking and your coordination will be diminished. If you immobilize your neck, as in wearing a stiff neck brace, after six weeks to two months, you will lose most if not all of these receptors. That is why proper treatment of your neck after trauma, as in an automobile accident, is vital for your best chance of recovery (discussed further later).

Mechanoreceptors are also located in ligaments. As you recall, ligaments are like tough rubber bands connecting two bones together at a joint. These ligaments allow joints and bones to move around each other while limiting excessive motion for protection. The mechanoreceptors monitor this motion through the ligaments.

I cannot stress enough the importance of these mechanoreceptors located in the ligaments and facet joints in the neck. Mechanoreceptors are located throughout the body, but by far the most densely populated area is the neck. The more distal, or farther away from the neck, the fewer mechanoreceptors will be found.

In the following chapters you will begin to understand how these mechanoreceptors can be causing your weird symptoms.

FIGURE 10

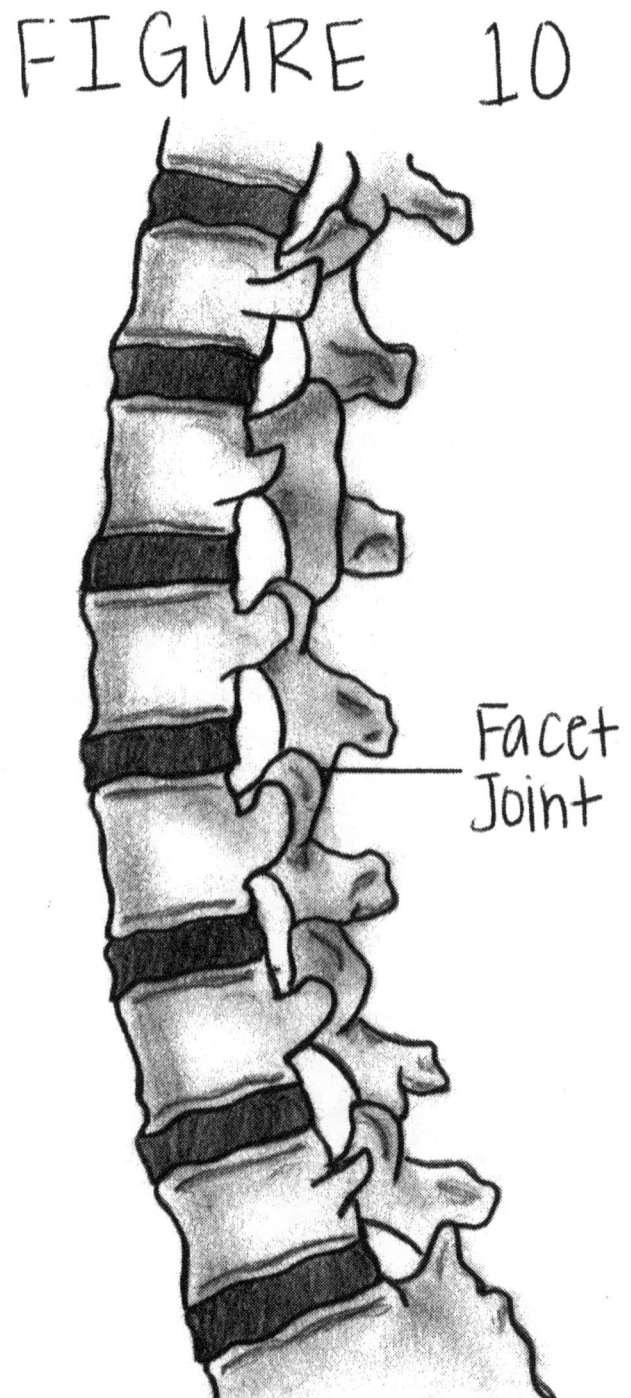

Facet Joint

DISCUSSION

As the spinal nerve exits your neck, it splits into two nerves. The Ventral Primary Rami goes to your arms, and the Dorsal Primary Rami goes back to your neck. These nerves in your neck monitor the movement of the bones in your neck. This is important for your survival if the bones move too excessively, damaging your spinal cord or vertebral artery. The nerves supply sensory supply, which is information going to the brain. The brain interprets the movement, and reacts with a motor response going back to the area. This response causes normal purposeful skilled movements if the motion is normal. If there is abnormal motion of the bones in your neck, the response to this could be leading to your symptoms.

CHAPTER IV

MECHANISM OF INJURY –
DAMAGING THE LIGAMENT

Recall in chapter two, we discussed how the ligaments in the body hold together, where two bones join together. These ligaments are like rubber bands, which are flexible, yet have tensile strength. The ligaments in your neck allow motion in your neck, yet limiting excessive motion.

Ligaments can be damaged by a number of different ways. If your ligaments are stretched slowly enough, your brain will react through the motor part of the nerve by recruiting muscles around the joint to help tighten and stabilize the joint. If the force stressing the joint is forceful enough, it will damage both the muscle and the ligament. If the joint is stressed too quickly for the muscles to help, and if the force is great enough, the ligaments will be damaged.

The most common cause of this situation is an accident such as an automobile accident. Previous studies indicated that it takes 125-215 milliseconds for a muscle to have enough time to help the ligament with support. However, during an automobile accident, stress was applied to the cervical joints in only 100 milliseconds, not giving the muscles enough time to help. The result is damaged, torn ligaments. Let us take a look at the results of a study involving a rear-end collision. [1]

Prior to impact, the neck has a normal C-curve. [Figure 11-A] When the vehicle is struck from behind, a series of events were noted in the cervical spine:

1. The lower neck and body were pushed forward with the head remaining. [Figure 11-B] This impact causes the lower neck to

go into forced extension (accentuated C-curve) and the upper neck in local flexion. The cervical spine assumes an abnormal S-curve.

2. The head will catch up with the body at approximately 100 ms by going into extension with the lower neck. [Figure 11-C] At this point, significant compression was noted at the posterior facet joint with anterior capsule tearing. [Figure 11-D]

Testing human volunteer rear-impacts revealed the time it takes for the muscles to respond to help is between 150-200ms. Therefore it is apparent in rear-end collisions, the muscles of the neck react too slowly to aid in protecting numerous structures in the cervical region which have the potential to serve as pain sources. This S-curve is not normal motion for the neck and if adequate force, the ligaments, limiting the motion of the bones in the neck, will be over-stressed and tearing will occur.

This tearing is known as a sprain (damaged ligaments). [Figure 12] The actual tearing of the ligaments in the neck is unique for each person. The ligament could possibly completely tear into two separate pieces. In reality, the usual damage is to separate collagen fibers within the ligament. [Figure 13] These tears within the ligament will cause the ligament to not be as stretchy as well as not as strong as it should be. This would allow the bones in your neck, specifically where this tear is, to move more than normal. This extra motion of the bones in your neck can cause all sorts of weird symptoms, and not just pain. Later we will explore how the extra motion of the bones disturb the mechanoreceptors of the Dorsal Rami branch of the neck spinal nerves lead to symptoms.

In my practice, there are a few points of interest that should be mentioned that have been revealed. If a person has a previous cervical fusion (two bones fused together), the accident will normally cause more damage to the joints of the two vertebrae directly above the fusion. For instance, if a person has fusion of C5/C6, if rear-ended, most ligament damage will usually occur at C4/C5 ligaments.

FIGURE 11

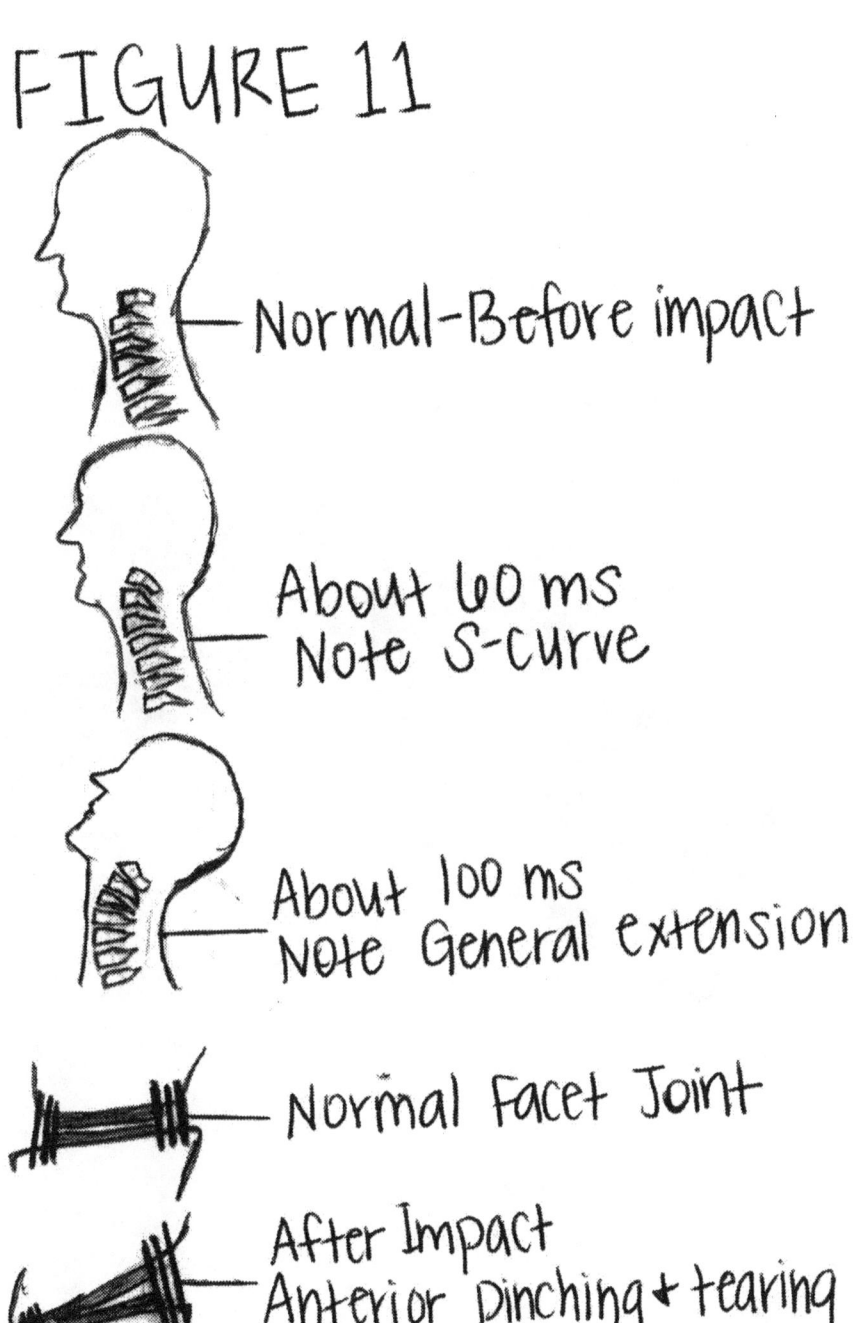

Normal-Before impact

About 60 ms
Note S-curve

About 100 ms
Note General extension

Normal Facet Joint

After Impact
Anterior pinching + tearing

FIGURE 12

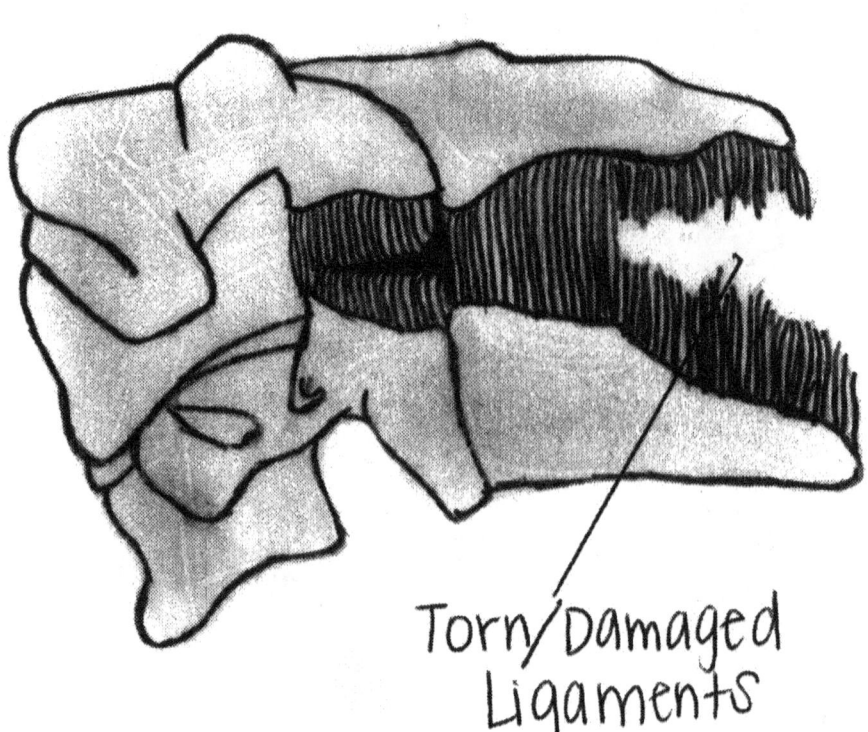

Torn/Damaged
Ligaments

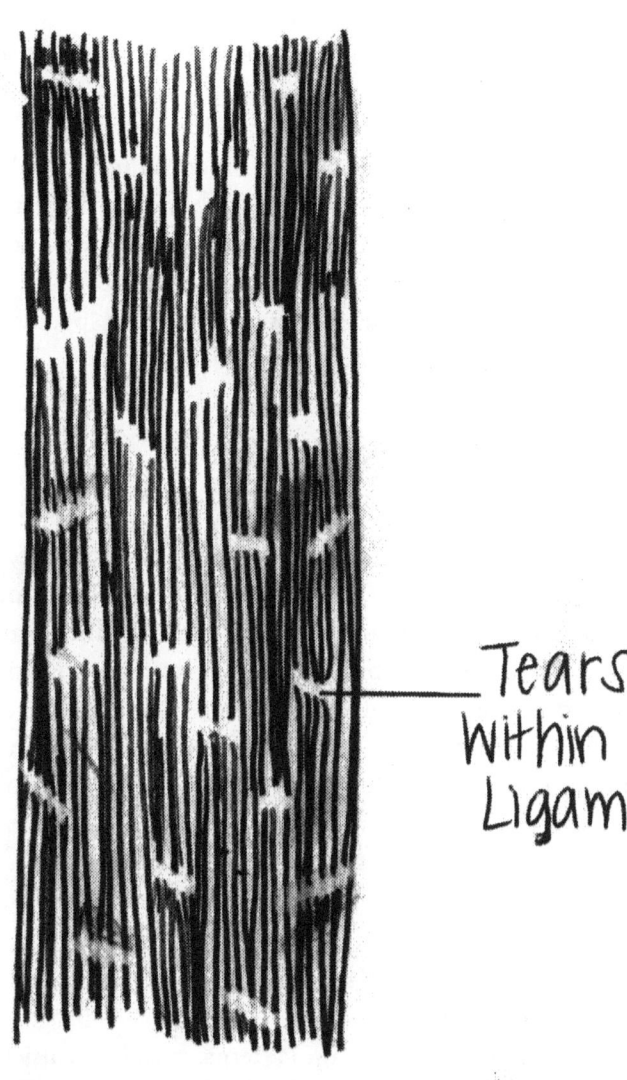

Tears
Within the
Ligament

FIGURE 13

If a person has any previous pathology in their neck which limits normal motion (degenerative disc disease, osteo-arthritis, etc.) the damage is usually more excessive immediately above this pathology. The specific ligament damaged and the severity of the tear is unique for each person, as well as several factors. For instance, if a person experiences a flexion/extension injury to his neck (rear-end collision) while he is looking to the right or left, this could tear the alar ligament. This ligament helps stabilize the top 2 neck bones during lateral bending and rotation. [Figure 14] This ligament could be torn on one side or both, which could lead to extra motion in this area. This would lead to symptoms coming from the nerve supplying this specific area, which monitors motion between C1/C2

SUMMARY

If a ligament is stretched too fast or with too much force, it will tear. In a typical rear end collision, the muscles do not have enough time to react to help support the ligaments. Once these ligaments are torn, they lose their strength and flexibility, allowing excessive motion between the specific bones they are stabilizing. This allows extra motion (hyper mobility) in the specific neck bones. When extra motion occurs, the specific nerve monitoring the specific area moving too much will be stimulated and the response will be discussed later.

(Endnotes)

[1] Kinematic Factors Influencing Pain Patterns, Joseph F. Cusick, md; Frank A Pintar, PhD; Harayon Yoganandan, PhD., From the Department of Neurosurgery, Medical college of Wisconsin, Spine 2001; 26:1252-1258 (June1, 2001).

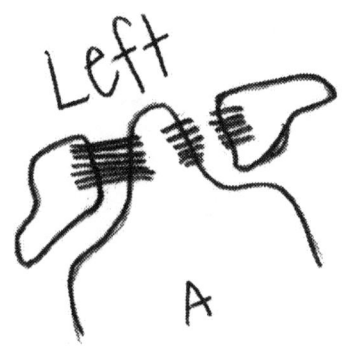

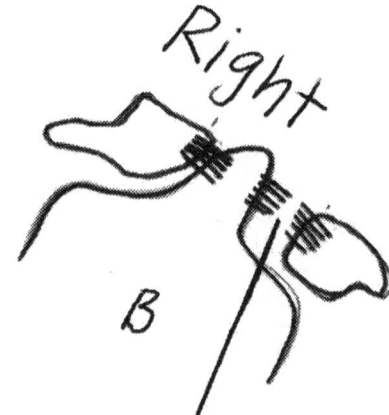

Torn Right Alar Ligament

NOTE: (B) A torn right alar ligament allows the atlas to slide on the axis to the right during right lateral bending.

(A) No sliding — Left alar ligament is intact.

FIGURE 14

Chapter V

Other Contributing Factors

In this chapter, several factors will be briefly discussed that someone would consider in determining the mechanism of injury.

An excellent start would be understanding that the degree of damage to a vehicle is not a predictor of outcome in determining occupant injury. There is evidence that duration of disability from whiplash is unrelated to the degree of trauma. "Our findings of no consistent association between physical factors, such as presence of a headrest or the degree of damage to the vehicle (assessed by whether the vehicle was drivable) are consistent with Stouner's conclusion that evidence for a causal link between trauma and chronic symptoms is sparse."[1,2] "The amount of damage sustained by the car bears little relationship to the force applied. To take an extreme example: If the car was stuck in concrete, the damage sustained might be very great, but the occupants would not be injured because the car could not move forward, where as, on ice, the damage to the car could be slight but the injuries sustained might be severe because of the rapid acceleration permitted."[3]

Acceleration of the occupant, or the degree of deceleration, is key in understanding injuries. Do you recall the documentary on television revealing different automobiles colliding with different structures at controlled speeds? These videos of the collisions were aimed at revealing to the consumer which automobile sustained less damage, which costs the consumer less to repair. After viewing this, a consumer would be led to believe that the vehicle that sustained the least damage would be the vehicle the consumer should own. The following research from engineers at the University of British Columbia is very interesting. They note the difference between a <u>plastic</u> vehicle and an <u>elastic</u> vehicle. A plastic vehicle is the one that sustains damage in the collision. An elastic vehicle is one that does not sustain damage in the collision. (Obviously we would assume the vehicle of choice is the elastic one). "The experimental results indicate that some vehicles can withstand a reasonably high speed impact without significant structural damage. The resulting occupant motions are marked by a lag interval, followed by a potentially dangerous acceleration up to speeds greater than that of the vehicle. For the occupant, the best ride down profile occurs when the vehicle behaves as a plastic body where larger deformations (vehicle damage) reduce the overall acceleration. To illustrate this concept, one particular vehicle tested at the UBC Accident Research facility showed no structural damage after a 15-km/h-barrier impact and was indicative of the fully elastic case. The overall change in velocity, delta V, experienced by the occupant in this vehicle would have been approximately 30 km/h due to the nearly equal and opposite rebound velocity, which resulted after the barrier impact. If this vehicle had behaved in a fully plastic manner upon impact, the same occupant would have experienced a delta V of only 15 km/h. Thus, based on an assumption of equal impact times during both collisions, the average acceleration experienced by the occupant in the elastic (no damage) vehicle would be approximately twice that of the plastic vehicle (damage vehicle). This theory implies that vehicles which do not sustain damage in low speed impacts can produce correspondingly higher dynamic loadings on their occupants that those which plastically deform under the same or possible more sever impact conditions." [4.]

Recall, in the previous chapter, we discussed that damaging the ligaments in the neck in an auto accident can be more severe if the occupant is unaware of the impact, not allowing enough time to recruit his surrounding voluntary (controlled) muscles. "The state of preparedness proved to be the first significant factor with respect to initial findings. Patients prepared for impact had a significantly lower frequency of multiple symptoms and lower intensity headaches." "Prepared occupants seemed to suffer less musculoskeletal strain." "Preparedness may also explain why whiplash syndrome rarely occurs in playing-field injuries, a part used (and misused) to stress psychological etiology. The state of preparedness has, to our knowledge, never been analyzed in previous clinical studies and certainly deserves attention in future research." [5.]

In a whiplash injury, the acceleration-deceleration movements of the neck are typically completed within 250 ms. The brevity of this period precludes any voluntary or reflex muscle response that might arrest, limit, or control the movements of a cervical motion segment. Without muscle control, the normal arcuate movement of a cervical motion segment must be disturbed, and the forces to which individual segments are subjected can be resisted only by passive ligamentous elements or bony contact. This sets the scene for a variety of possible injuries. [6.]

If the occupant's head is turned (rotated) during the impact, this increases the risk of injury. "Injuries are greater when nonsymmetrical loads are implied to the spine. This occurs when the spine sustains a rotary injury. The injuries are increased because the facet joints lockout spinal motion, making the neck rigid, less resilient, and more susceptible to injury. When the head is rotated 45 degrees to one side, the amount of extension that side of the spine is capable of is decreased by 50%. This results in increased compressive loads on the facet joints, articular pillars on the ipsilateral side, and increased tensor loads at the facet joints on the contralateral side. The intervertebral foramen are smaller on the side of rotation and lateral flexion, and the neurovascular bundles are more vulnerable to compressive injuries." [7.] If the occupant in an accident has pre-existing degenerative joint disease, the injury and expected time of recovery are both increased. When normal spinal motion is limited due to degenerative arthritic changes, acceleration energy could not be dispersed equally. "With advancing age, especially in the presence of degenerative disease, the tissues become inelastic and are easily torn." [8.]

"The films should be inspected especially for evidence of pre-existing structural changes or for alteration, which are frequently associated with a more difficult, more prolonged, and less complete recovery. These changes may include the presence of osteophytes, foraminal encroachment on the oblique projections, and the presence of intervertebral disc space narrowing. When hyperextension injury occurs in the presence of pre-existing osteophyte formation, there is further narrowing of the spinal canal, which increase the potential for injury to the nerve roots or cord." [9.]

This may explain why in clinical settings, when reviewing damage to the cervical spine with someone who had previous cervical fusion (surgical or congenital), the ligament damage is more severe usually at the joints directly above the fusion. This damage can be confirmed through dynamic motion x-ray studies, followed by review of this patients scleratome patterns.

(Endnotes)

[1] Richard Townsend Gun, SS, FAFOM, Orso Lorenzo Osti, MD, PhD, FRACS, FAOrthA, Alison O'Riordon, MPhil, Freddie Mpelasoka, PhD, and James Farrell Smyth, BAO, FACEM, FFAEM, FRCSI, DCH, BA - Risk Factors for Prolonged Disability after Whiplash Injury: A Prospective Study. Spine Volume 30, Number 4, pp 386-391.

[2] Stourner L.J The Nasologic Status of Whiplash Syndrome: A critical review. Spine 1996; 21: 2735-46

[3] Macnab, in The Spine, Saunders, 1982, pg. 648.

[4] Navin, F., M. Macnab, et al. (1989). An Investigation into Vehicle and Occupant Response Subjected to Low-Speed Rear Impact. Proceedings of the Multidisciplinary Road Safety Conference VI, June 5-7, 1989, Frederiction, New Brunswick, Canada.

[5] Sturzenegger, M., G. Distafano, et al. (1994) "Presenting Symptoms and Signs After Whiplash Injury: The Influence of Accident Mechanism." Neurology 44: 688-93.

[6] Lord, in Spine: State of the Art Reviews: Cervical Flexion-Extension/ Whiplash Injuries, Hanley & Belfus, Sept. 1993, pg. 374.

[7] Hausy, Whiplash Injuries of the Cervical Spine and Their Clinical Seaquelae, AM Journal of Pain Management, January, 1994.

[8] Turek, Orthopedics Principle and their Applications, Lippincott, 1977 pg. 740.

[9] Hirsh, Whiplash Syndrome Fact or Fiction? Orthopedic Clinics of North America, Oct. 1988.

CHAPTER VI

YOUR BODY'S RESPONSE
(TO A DAMAGED LIGAMENT)

Ligaments are comprised of many collagen fibers (triple-helix structure with intertwining cross-links) interweaving with fibrous bundles, which increase the structural stability and elasticity. In an automobile accident, the most common ligament damage occurs inside the ligament structure, and not complete tearing. "It is incredible how this complex structure is laid down and reinforced in direct response to the exact stresses applied to it" (Boyd's pathology). In other words, the direction of the fiber formation appears to be dependent directly upon the angle of the stress applied to it. (Note this will be a very important treatment consideration). This capability of a ligament to directly form itself as a result of the stresses applied to it gives the ligament not only more tensile strength, but also the ability to stretch and recoil. If parts of a ligament structure are damaged, it is crucial the ligament heals with the original normal collagen fibers and inter-twined elastin forming its original normal structure. If the body's reaction to ligament damage is known, then the treatment of this damaged area is better understood.

The body's reaction following a damaged torn ligament has several phases, which overlap considerably. An initial response will be discussed using Guyton's Textbook of Medical Physiology.

"The process of inflammation is the body's first response to tissue (ligament) damage. It is made up of sequential steps taking place. When tissue injury occurs, whether it is caused by bacteria, trauma, chemicals, heat, or any other phenomenon, large quantities of histamine, bradykinin, serotonin, and other substances are liberated by the damaged tissue into the surrounding fluid. These, especially the histamine, increase the local blood flow allowing large quantities of fluid and protein to initiate the healing process. White blood cells invade the area for defense against any invading bacteria or other foreign substances. Macrophages phagocytize (engulf) bacteria and necrotic (dead) tissue cells in the area." This increases blood flow to the damaged area causing localized swelling and redness. This process will also irritate the local sensory nerve fibers, leading to pain and localized muscle spasms. This reaction is your body's way of informing you not to use the damaged area for protection from further damage. This inflammation process is vital to clean out torn, dead debris and to initiate the necessary events that heal the damaged area. A key cell that migrates to the area is known as the fibroblast. Fibroblasts are very active during repair of your body's damaged tissue. They multiply to produce large numbers of cells to fill in the vacant torn, damaged areas in the ligament. This process is like putting a patch over the damaged area. Fibroblasts have an extremely unique capability of differentiating into three different main mature cells. They are:

1. Collagenoblast- leading to the original collagen fibers replacing the torn tissue.
2. Chondroblast- leading to scar tissue.
3. Osteoblast- leading to hard, calcified bone cells.

Obviously, our desire is to have the fibroblast turn into normal ligament tissue. This stretchy, tensile strong ligament would allow the bones it supports to move normally. If scar tissue replaces the torn fibers, the bones' movement would be restricted, thereby irritating the sensory nerves supplying the area and leading to unwanted symptoms. Another problem that occurs frequently is not enough fibroblasts differentiating in the area, leading to the ligament not being able to restrict the bones enough. In other words, the bones would be hypermobile, moving too much. This would also irritate the sensory nerve fibers, leading to unwanted symptoms.

As these fibroblasts cover the damaged area, they actually have specialized contractile fibroblasts (myofibroblasts) that shorten and try to bring the ligament to original length.

Would it not be nice if we could influence the fibroblast to:

1. line up the new fibers in the same direction the initial fibers lined up.
2. replace the damaged cells with original collagen fibers.
3. return the ligament to its original length.

This will be discussed in treatment considerations.

CHAPTER VII

MOST COMMON SYMPTOMS (FOLLOWING DAMAGED CERVICAL LIGAMENTS)

In this chapter, and the following few chapters on other symptoms, The Neck Step will attempt to explain the actual cause of the most common symptoms following an automobile accident.

The following is a result of a study on 41 patients complaining with neck pain. Also associated with their symptoms included:

Headache	88%
Disturbance of memory and/or concentration	71%
Paresthesia in upper limb	68%
Weakness/heaviness in arms	68%
Dizziness	53%
Visual disturbances	42%

39.6% of those injured in a rear-end auto accident have chronic neck pain, even after 7 years. [1.]

Symptoms of chronic whiplash include:
1. Cervical pain
2. Headache
3. Cognitive difficulties
4. Visual disturbances
5. Dizziness [2.]

In order to understand how it is possible for symptoms, such as those above, as a result of an auto accident; we first need to be familiar with the nerves in the neck that cause these symptoms. There are four types of nerves that supply the neck for sensory.

Type I- Corpuscles, located in fibrous capsule at junction of synovial tissue- not in synovial tissue.
- Low threshold- if tension, continuous firing persists even if immobile- if not in resting potential.
- Biggest contribution in accuracy of control mechanoreceptors

Type II- Corpuscles in synovial joints, at junction of fibrous capsule
- Low threshold -quick firing- short- not fire if immobile - only at initial movement
- Always motor response
- Mechanoreceptors

Type III - Corpuscles in ligaments
- High threshold - continuous firing if tension remains high, located at attachments
- Don't fire with minor/moderate tension
- Mechanoreceptors

Type IV - Nociceptive (pain receptors)
- In joint capsules, ligament (throughout entire ligament) and tendon.
- Free nerve endings, unmyelinated throughout entire ligament
- In fibrous capsules- unmyelinated that weaves through the entire joint capsule.

Note- when a joint is immobile, there is tonic static discharge from Type I receptor. When you stretch a joint, Type I is augmented and returned to normal discharge when at resting position. Type II receptors emits only a very brief discharge at change of tension. They don't fire during immobilization.

Type I receptors are relayed throughout the central nervous system, where they make major contribution to postural sensation, one's conscious awareness of the static position of one's joints and to kinesthesis (one's conscious assessment of the direction, velocity, and amplitude of joints' movement), generally, actively, and passively. If you take a normal subject, anesthetize the joint capsule- their capacity to recognize accurately the static position of that joint with their eyes closed and their capacity to the amplitude and velocity of an imposed joint movement is very grossly impaired, but not completely abolished. If mechano-receptors destroyed, as in osteo-arthritis, rheumatoid arthritis, or destroyed by direct trauma (auto-accident), then all such patients show impairment of postural sensation and of kinesthesis related to the affected joint.

The most important regulators of balance are from the mechano-receptors in the cervical spine. Far more input than from the vestibular system. In normal cervical spine mechano-receptors, it can compensate totally for an absolute vestibular deficit. No disturbance of posture, gait, and conscious awareness of balance. If altered or deficient cervical mechano-receptors - total compensation of vestibular system is impossible. Discharges from the cervical mechano-receptors, particularly those from the upper 4, are transmitted cephalad (above) to the motor neuron pools of the eye muscles, jaw muscles, and to the tongue musculature. This explains why after events such as whiplash, the patients show disturbance of eye movements, disturbance of speech articulation, disturbance of balance, posture, and gait and sometimes problems while chewing. This syndrome is usually blamed on vestibular damage or to inadequate blood flow in the basilar artery." -Dr. Barry Wyke- Director of the Neurological unit for the Royal College of Surgeons in England.

Those nerves described above are the types of nerves found in your neck. The first three types can cause symptoms of dizziness, blurred vision, loss of balance/coordination, etc. Irritation of type 4 will cause pain. This pain can be localized to the damaged area, but it is usually also referred somewhere else. This is known as a sclerotome.

Sclerotome pain patterns are tremendously overlooked and probably the single-most reason someone is reading this book. They are hurting and having weird symptoms and no one can explain why. Recall when the spinal nerve exits the cervical spine; it splits into two different nerves: The Ventral Rami and the Dorsal Rami. [Figure 15] The Ventral Rami of the lower cervical segments innervate (go into) the arms. These nerves are easily tested to determine any problems. (EMG, deep tendon reflex, pinwheel sensory exam, specific muscle test, etc.)

The Dorsal Rami innervates the posterior areas of the spine. When these nerves are irritated, they refer pain. These nerves are difficult to test in isolation. Rarely will you find a physician diagnose this problem for two main reasons. The first reason is these sclerotome pain patterns cannot be objectively confirmed by independent test. The second reason is this referral pain source is not well understood by most physicians.

The idea that pain could be perceived at a site distant from its source has confused many patients and led to many a misinterpretation by physicians. Patients may lead the unwary physician away from the site of true pathology because they believe the pain to originate in a painful (but clinically and physiologically normal) distant site. [3.]

Recall in chapter 2, we learned there are seven cervical neck vertebra and from above and below each vertebra, exits a nerve. There are eight of these nerves. [Figure 16] If you are experiencing referred achy pain (sclerotome), the following specific list of where each of the eight nerves go will help you understand where your pain can be coming from.

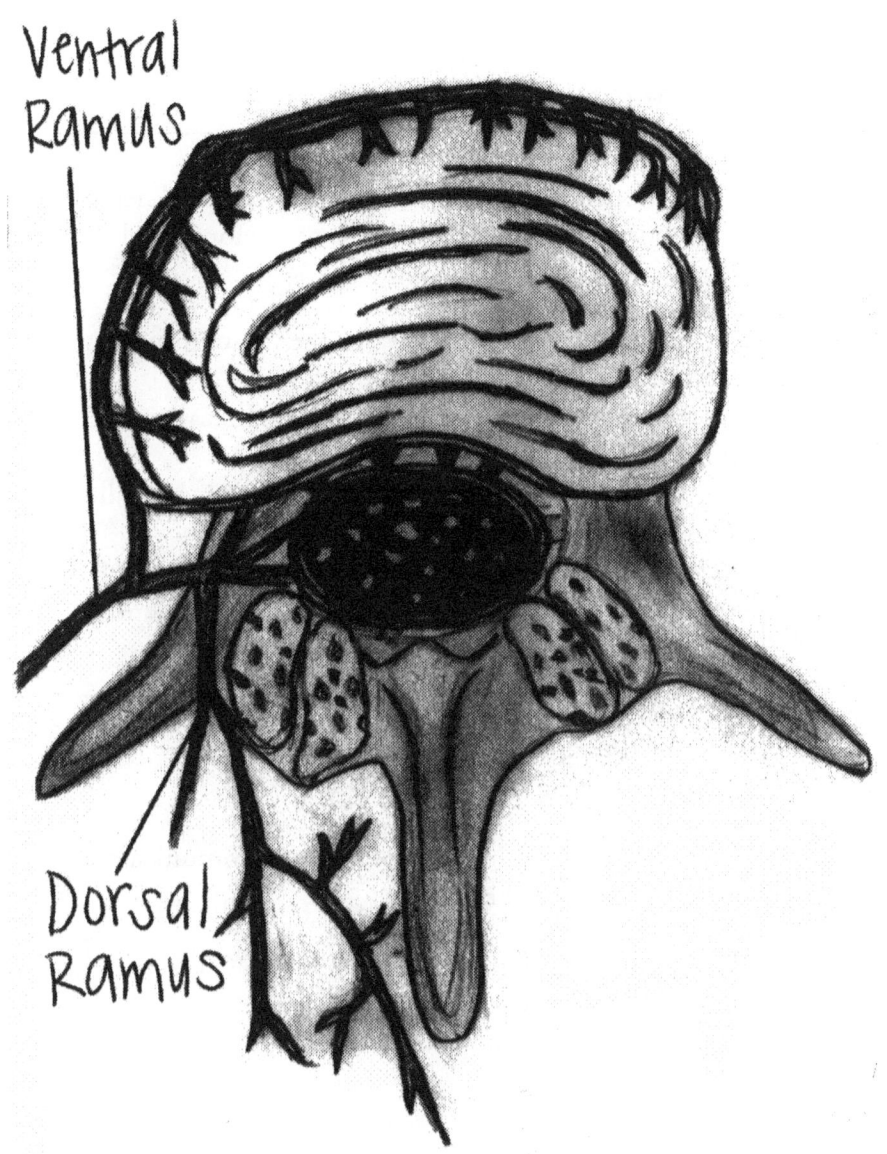

Ventral Ramus

Dorsal Ramus

FIGURE 15

Nerve	Area it goes into (innervates)
C1	1). Sub-occipital muscles 2). Communicating branch with C2
C2	1). Medial branch-greater occipital nerve -Communicating branch for the third occipital nerve -Inserts into the trapezius and sternocleidomastoid -Innervates the occipital skin 2). Lateral branch- passes above the mastoid process and behind the pinna (ear) -Communicates with the third cervical dorsal ramus 3). Intermediate branch- runs rostrally and vertically across the top of the skull with branches of the occipital artery- as far as the coronal suture communicates with the terminal branches of the supraorbital nerve.
	4). Specific branches to the occipital artery, the superficial temporal artery, and the posterior surface of the auricle (flap of the ear). 5). Superior communicating branch- communicates with the first dorsal ramous 6). Inferior communicating branch- C2/C3 facet joints (meets the third cervical dorsal ramous).

C3	1). Medial branch (third occipital nerve). -superior facet C3 -Communicates with the greater and lesser occipital nerve -trapezious -Supplies the skin over the rostral end of the neck and occiput below the external occipital protuberance. -uppermost fibers of the multifidus -C2/C3 facet joint
C 4 - C8	1). Lateral branch- (C4-C7) -Longissmus cervicis and splenius Cervicis muscles C8- ilio costalis cervicis 2). Medial branch- multifidus -Each nerve exclusively innervates those fibers that attach to the spinous process with a segmental number one less that that of the nerve. E.g. C4 medial branch innervates those fibers that attach to the C3 spinous process. -innervates the trapezius -Facet joint above and to below that medial branch -Articular branches from adjacent levels may communicate with one another to form a communicating loop dorsal to the facet joint. [Figure 17 & 18]

Note: occiput/atlas and lateral atlas/axis are not innervated by the dorsal rami. The C2 dorsal ramus runs dorsally and caudally well away from the joint. Occiput/Atlas, atlas/axis are innervated by ventral rami.

Noxious stimulation (damage/trauma to the area) of the muscle supplied by the C1 and C2 dorsal rami can produce referred pain to the head (relates to suboccipital trigger points and headaches).

Understanding the above nerve innervations from the spine, you can basically locate your possible problem by tracing from your aching pain area back to the spinal nerve source. For instance, if you are experiencing headaches going from the back of your head (occiput) to the front above your eye (supraorbital), it is very possible your nerve problem could be the medial and intermediate branch from C2 nerve. If your neck has been through trauma in the past, for instance an automobile accident, then you could possibly have ligament damage near the C2 nerve, causing the bones to move extra, irritating this nerve. Are you starting to get the whole picture or idea? The trauma to your neck could have been very recent. For some unknown reason, many of my patients start having headaches (noticeably worse) following at ten years after the accident.

If you are experiencing achy pains, referred to a generally specific area, try and trace the ache back to its possible cervical nerve.

(Endnotes)

[1] Chronic Cervical Zygopophyseal Joint Pain after Whiplash, Spine 1996; 21: 1737-1744 (August)

[2] KINEMATIC FACTORS INFLUENCING PAIN PATTERNS, Spine 2001; 26: 1252-1258 (June 1, 2001)

[3] Referred Pain Syndromes of the Head and Neck, Physical Medicine and Rehabilitation: State of the Art Reviews – Vol 5, No. 3, October 1991 Philadelphia, Hanley, and Belfus, Inc.

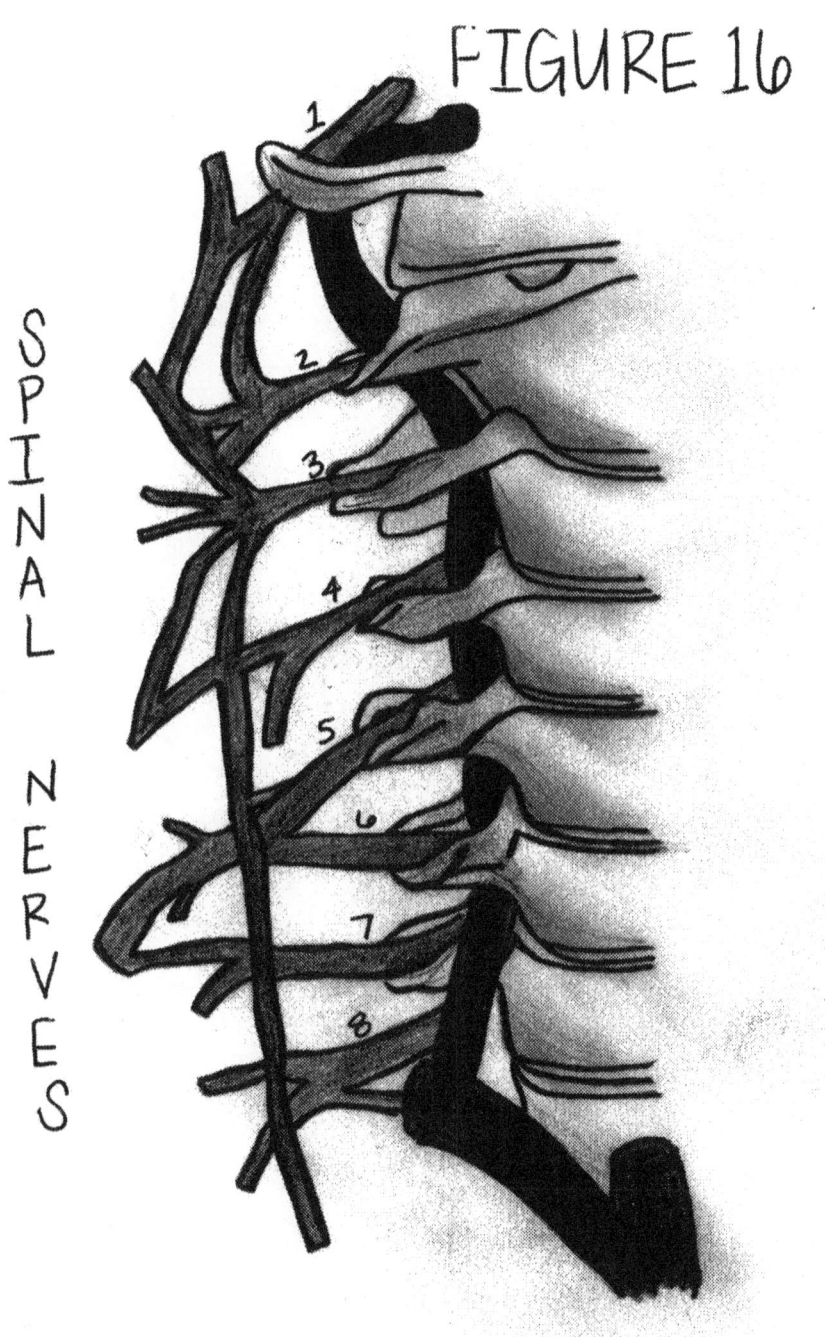

FIGURE 16

SPINAL NERVES

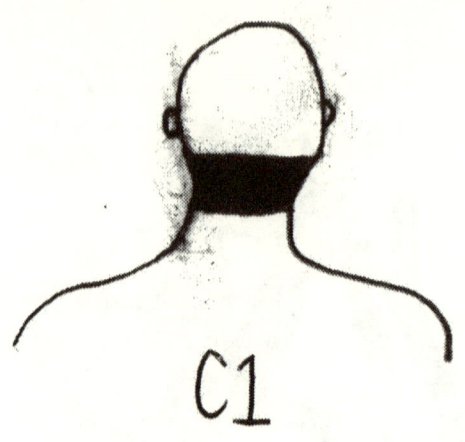

C1

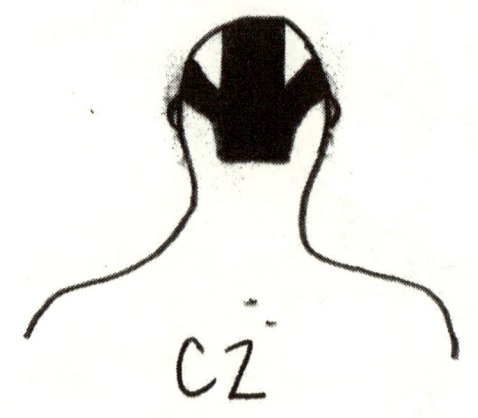

C2

FIGURE 17

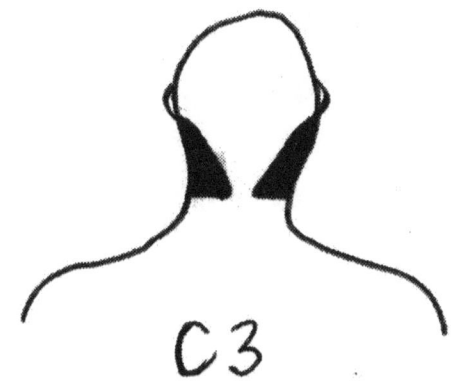

C3

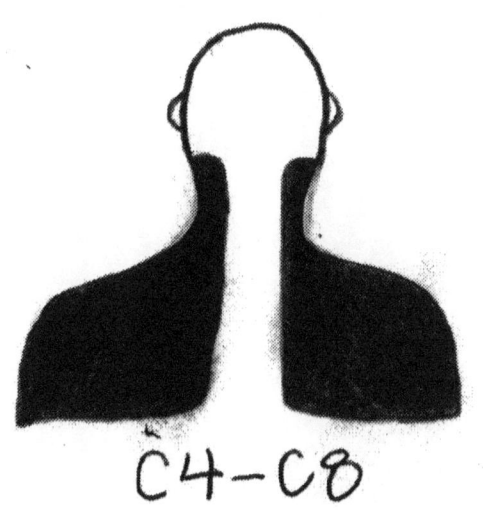

C4-C8

FIGURE 18

Chapter VIII

Neck Pain

Do you ever wonder why your neck is hurting? Where is the pain actually coming from?

In this chapter, we will review two key sources of neck pain. Before we look at where these sources could be causing you neck pain, let's first understand how pain is perceived. Pain, or the sensation of pain, is carried from the body to the brain by nociceptive nerve fibers. According to Dorland's medical dictionary, nociceptor is a receptor that is stimulated by injury; a receptor for pain. If you perceive pain, these nociceptor fibers carry the sensation in your body. Dr. Barry Wyke tells us "pain is an unpleasant emotional disorder evoked by sufficient activity in the nociceptive system. The nociceptive receptor systems may be irritated by sufficient mechanical distortion of a tissue, or it may be irritated by the exposure of the unmyelinated nerve fibers to depolarizing agents concentrating in the inter-structural fluids bathing these unmyelinated nerve fibers. Differential diagnosis should be one of these two (mechanical or chemical), or it is a combination of both. If you squeeze, stretch, or cut nerve fibers, you depolarize them.

What are the chemical causes of pain? These agents depolarize the nerves, (which mean they are a possible chemical source of pain).

Weakest	o Lactic acid
↓	o Potassium ions
↓	o 5-hydroxytryptomine
↓	o Kinins – (produced by breakdown of cellular proteins)
↓	
↓	
↓	o Proteins – (released from damaged tissue)
↓	
↓	o Prostoglandin
Strongest	o Histamine

In lactic acid or potassium ions - released from ischemic tissue as in muscular pain fatigue. That's why atherosclerotic valve vessels produce pain in the middle of the night- exercise, stretching, or massage relieves the pain. This accelerates venous drainage. Prostaglandins are from dying, necrosed, or traumatized cells. The other four raise inflammatory responses."

The ligaments and tendons in your neck have these nociceptive nerve fibers. Therefore, if your muscles in your neck are strained or if the ligaments in your neck are sprained, the inflammatory response, reacting to this trauma, will stimulate these nociceptive sensory fibers, giving you the sensation of pain. This would be an example of chemical nociceptive stimulation. Pain coming from physical and chemical nociceptive stimulation may be coming from two keys areas in your neck, the facet joints, and/or your intervertebral disc. [figure 19] Following an auto accident, cervical facet joint pain is the most common source of persistent chronic pain. [1]

In order for an area in the body to be capable of producing pain, free nerve endings of pain (nociceptive) fibers must be present. In the cervical spine, not only do you have these free nerve endings located in the facet joint, but you also have mechanoreceptors (proprioceptive) nerve fibers as well. [2]

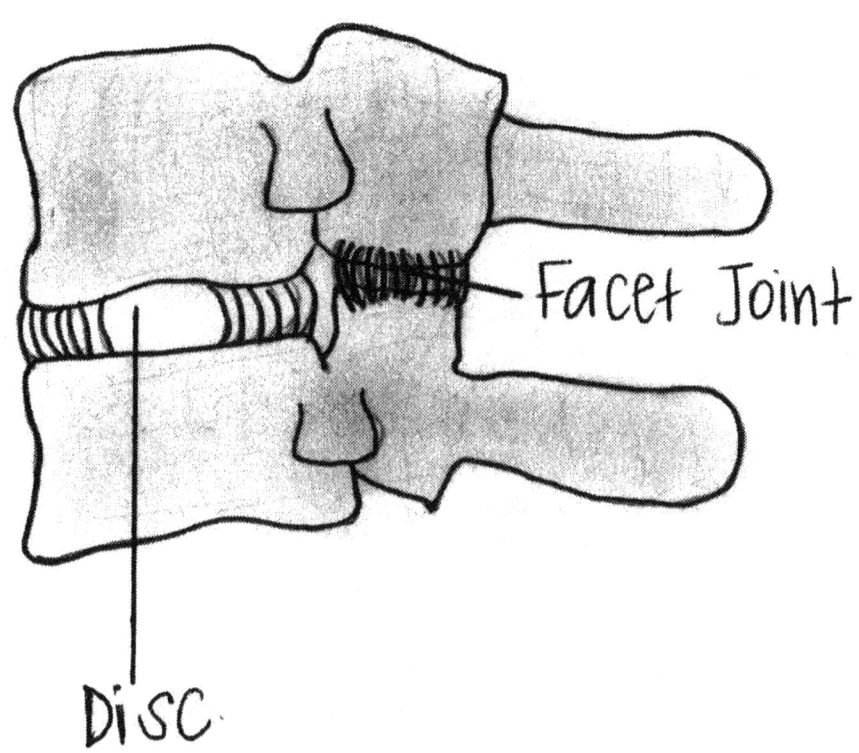

Facet Joint

Disc

FIGURE 19

If you recall in chapter IV mechanism of injury, during a typical auto accident, the cervical spine is forced into a s-shaped curve instead of the normal c-curve. This stress of these joints exceeds their physiologic motion limits. [3] Therefore, if the stress is too far on these joints, the ligaments holding these joints together are over-stretched and torn. This would allow excessive motion of these facet joints irritating both the mechanoreceptor (proprioceptive) and pain (nociceptive) nerve fibers in the cervical facet joints. The conclusion of these studies reveals there is a high probability if you have chronic neck pain, following an injury, as in an automobile accident, the pain is coming from your cervical facet joints.

According to some authors, they noted that experiments on healthy volunteers indicate that during the rear end collision, when the trunk is forced upwards toward the head, and the cervical spine goes into the unnatural "s" shape – "During this motion, at about 100 milliseconds after impact, the lower cervical vertebrae undergo extension but without translation. This motion causes the vertebral bodies to separate anteriorly and the zygapophysial (facet) joints to impact posteriorly. The lesions are likely to result from such motions as tears of the anterior annulus fibrosis (disc injury), and fractures or contusions of the zygapophyseal (facet) joints. These are the lesions found post mortem in victims of fatal motor vehicle crashes." [4] [Figure 20}

FIGURE 20

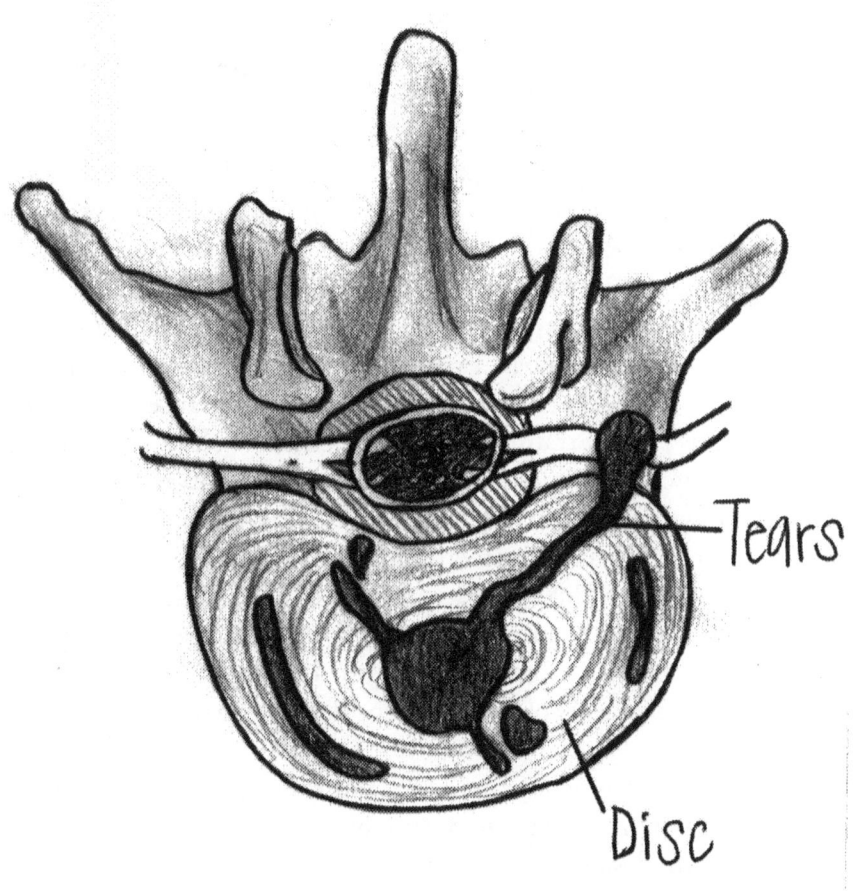

Tears

Disc

They also noted:

1) Facet joint pain is the single most common basis for chronic neck pain after whiplash, accounting for at least 50%, and up to 80% of patients pain.

2) The segmental levels most commonly involved are C5-6 and C2-3.

3) In patients with chronic headache as the dominant complaint after whiplash, the source of pain can be traced to the C2-3 facet joint in approximately 53% of cases.

Just to add from this study a few additional unique remarks:

Mental (psychological) stress/distress following automobile accidents is common, "However, psychosocial factors do not cause neck pain, nor are they predictive of chronicity." "Rather, psychological distress is secondary to chronic pain. If pain is completely relieved, psychological distress disappears. If the pain recurs, psychological distress reappears, but is removed if pain is once again relieved."

Now, back to what causes the neck pain following trauma, as in a rear-end collision. Studies indicate that the impact from behind deforms the cervical spine in a way that the force stresses and damages structures in the neck. The single most common cause of neck pain following this type of trauma is the facet joints. [5] Keep in mind when the neck is forced in hyperextension, the superior area of the facets are displaced downward to an extreme degree, and the ligaments around the facet joints (capsular ligaments) are stretched. [6]

"In studies in which experimental animals or cadavers have been subjected to whiplash motion, injuries to the cervical zagapophyseal joints are among the most common and consistent lesion produced. The lesions include tears of the joint capsules, intraarticular hemorrhage and impaction fractures."

"Postmortem studies of victims of motor vehicle accidents reveal that zygapophyseal joint injuries are common, being present in 86% of necks examined. The lesions include capsular tears, rupture of meniscoids, intraarticular hemorrhage, and small fractures. [7]

The studies are numerous documenting during trauma to your neck, as in an automobile rear-end collision, damage, over-stressed, torn capsular (facet) ligaments are a major cause for your pain.

Probably the second most overlooked and misunderstood cause of your neck pain could be coming from the cushion (fibro-cartilage) between the bones in your neck, called intervertebral disc. For a structure in your neck, such as an intervertebral disc, to be considered as a possible pain source, it must meet the following criteria.

1) Does the intervetebral disc contain nociceptive (pain) sensory nerve fibers to send pain signals?
2) During trauma to the neck, as in a rear-end collision, are the intervertebral disc stressed physically enough to damage their structure firing their nociceptive fibers causing pain?

When most people think of a disc problem, they immediately picture a ruptured (herniated) disc pressing on a nerve causing pain. This is a common problem in low back injuries. However, "more recently, postmortem studies have found that after whiplash injuries, ligamentous injuries are extremely common in the cervical spine and that herniation of the nucleus pulposus is a rare event." [8.] If that is the case, what actually happens to a disc during injury to actually cause the neck pain?

First, the question of whether intervertebral disc have an innervation has long been a subject of contention. In other words, does the cervical intervetebral disc have nociceptive fibers in the disc, which if damaged, would be a source of pain itself? Or does a disc have to rupture, and press on a nerve, outside the disc itself, to cause any pain? This is a very important concept for you to understand. Once again, can damage inside a disc cause pain? Can a disc be a source of pain all by itself? The answer is simple. The cervical intervertebral disc have nociceptive pain fibers located inside their structure. [Figure 21]

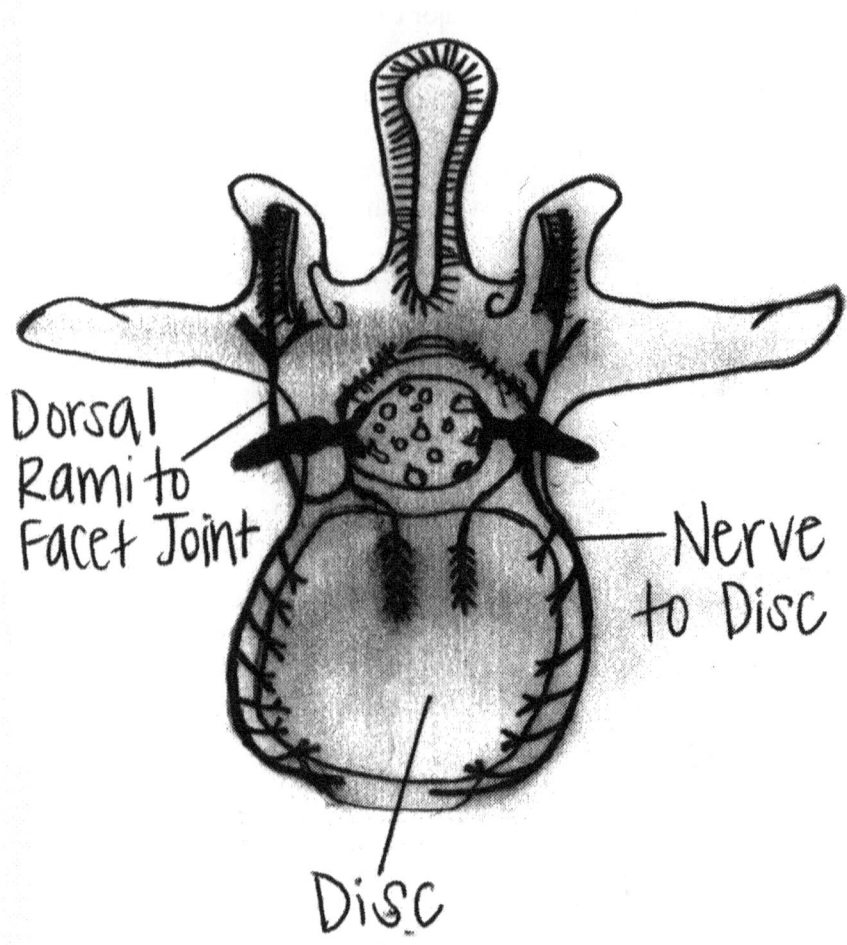

Dorsal Rami to Facet Joint

Nerve to Disc

Disc

FIGURE 21

"In summary, the present study has established that the cervical sinuvertebral nerves have a course and distribution analogous to those in the lumbar region, and that these nerves, together with branches of the vertebral nerve, supply the cervical intervertebral discs." [9.]

Therefore, since the cervical intervertebral disc does contain nociceptive (pain) fibers, if it is injured, it can be a source of pain itself. Why is this possibly extremely important to you? This could be your problem, a damaged cervical intervetebral disc causing your neck pain. But you state that's impossible because you had x-rays, a cat scan, and a MRI of your neck and they told you everything, including your disc, were normal. Guess what? When a physician orders a MRI/Cat Scan of the disc, most of the time, they are looking for a disc protrusion, protruding out far enough to put direct pressure on the ventral primary rami nerve. Rare, extremely rare, is a disc, by itself, considered a pain source. If the annulus fibrosus (circular fibers of a disc surrounding the nucleus) are torn or damaged, their nociceptive (pain) fibers will cause neck pain. [Figure 22]

Can trauma to your neck, such as an automobile accident, cause tears of your disc in your cervical spine? During a rear-end collision, the neck is compressed together, with compressive force as much as 500-600 pounds. [10.] Damage to the cervical intervertebral disc have been reported from several sources." It has been suggested that anterior tears could result from the nucleus pulposus bursting through the anterior annulus after being compressed by the extension of the motion segment." [11.]

FIGURE 22

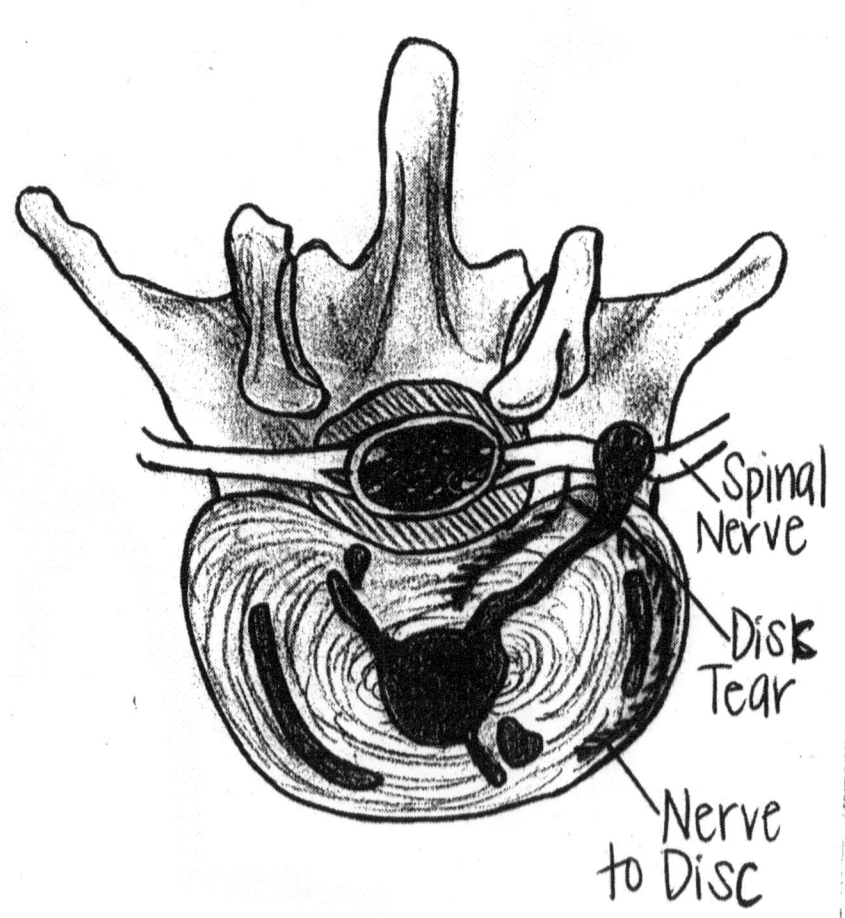

Spinal Nerve

Disk Tear

Nerve to Disc

"That the cervical discs can intrinsically be a source of pain has been a contentious issue. Reservations have been based on the impression that these structures lacked a nerve supply. It is now evident, however, that these discs are well endowed with a nerve supply anteriorly, posterolaterally, and posteriorly, and therefore must be regarded as potential sources of pain. The sources of neck pain are the muscles, joints, and intervertebral discs of the neck. Disc pain probably results from strain or tears of the annulus fibrosus." [12]

(Endnotes)

[1] THE PREVALENCE OF CHRONIC CERVICAL ZYGAPOPHYSIAL JOINT PAIN AFTER WHIPLASH. Barnsley L. Lord SM, Wallis BJ, Bogduk N Spine 1995 Jan 1;20 (1): 20-5

[2] MECHANORECEPTOR ENDINGS IN HUMAN CERVICAL FACET JOINTS. Robert f. McLain, MD SPINE Volume 19, Number 5, pp 495-501 (MARCH 1 1994)

[3] Graur, J.N., M.M. Panjabi, et. Al, (1997). "Whiplash produces a s-shaped curvature of the neck with hyperextension at lower levels." Spine 22 (21): 2489-94

[4] Controversies in Neurology Whiplash, The Evidence for AN ORGANIC Etiology. Arch Neurol, Vol. 57 No.4, April 2000, 590-91 Nikolai Bogduk, MD, PhD, D Sci Robert Teasell, M.D. FRCPC

[5] Biomechanics of the Cervical Spine Part 3: minor injuries. Clin Biomech 2001 May; 16 (4): 267-75

[6] Turek, Orthopaedics, Lippincott, 1977, p. 740

[7] Lord, in Spine: State of the Art Reviews: Cervical Flexion – Extension/ Whiplash Injuries, Hanley and Belfus, Sept. 1993, p. 362

[8] The ligaments and Anulus Fibrosus of Human Adult Cervical Intervertebral Discs Susan Mercer, B. Phty (Hons), msc, PhD, and Nikolai Bogduk, MD, PhD, DSC, FAFRMT

[9] The Innervation of the Cervical Intervertebral Discs NIKOLAI BOGDUK, BSC (Med), MB BS, PhD, Morgan Windsor, B Med Sci, and Adam Inglis, Bmed Scie, Spine. Volume 13. Number 1. 1988

[10] Calliet, Neck And Arm Pain. DAVIS Company, 1981 p. 81

[11] Barnsley, in Spine: State of the Art Reviews: Cervical Flexion – Extension/ Whiplash Injuries, Hanley and Belfus, Sept. 1993 p. 334-335

[12] Neck Pain: an update. Nikolai Bogduk Australian Family Physician Vol 17. No.2 February 1988. pp. 75-80

Chapter IX

Headaches

Understanding where your headaches are coming from is the goal of this chapter.

In most cases, headaches are not signs of a serious, life-threatening problem. However, if you are experiencing a sudden onset of headaches, which started for no apparent reason, they may disturb you while sleeping or active and nothing you take or do will relieve them, please seek a neurological consultation to rule out serious pathologies.

Based on the National Headache Foundation, more than 45 million Americans suffer from headaches, and many report pain and associated symptoms of this disease can be so severe that their ability to perform normal work, school, family, and social activities are impacted. In fact, industry loses approximately 50 billion per year due to absenteeism, lost productivity, and medical expenses caused by a headache. In excess of 4 billion dollars are spent annually on over-the-counter pain relievers for headaches. Many of these are ineffective for the headache sufferer.

Chronic headache sufferers should be aware of a phenomenon known as REBOUND HEADACHES. Taking medication each day for headaches may lead to more frequent and more severe headaches. Rebound headaches usually occur in the mornings or when you miss a dose of medication that you take regularly. As your nervous system withdraws from the lack of your instant-relief medicine, your headaches will occur sooner due to the withdrawal and not the initial cause of your headaches. This keeps you on a vicious cycle caused by the pain meds, or lack of them, if taken for weeks or longer in some cases. Discontinued use of your quick fix pain meds are the only solution. However, sudden withdrawal of even over-the-counter meds may be dangerous. If you believe you may be suffering from Rebound Headaches, please consult your physician for appropriate tapering off of your meds.

Here is a very important question I would like you to ponder over a few minutes. Is the treatment for your headaches only treating your symptoms, or is the focus of your treatment aimed at eliminating the actual cause of your headaches? Understanding where your headaches are coming from is the goal of this chapter.

There are many causes of headaches. The most common type is known as Tension-Type Headaches. Their symptoms are dull-pressure like pain, worse in the scalp, temples, or base of the neck, tight band or vise on the head. Most causes of headaches actually originate in the patients neck. The damaged area is located in the cervical spine (neck) and pain (sclerotome pattern) is perceived or felt in the head. This is a common occurrence when your body refers pain from one area to another. An example of this sclerotome pain is when someone has a heart attack. American Heart Association teaches us that if someone is having a heart attack, pain may be felt in the jaw, down one or both arms, etc.. There is no damage to the tissue to cause pain in these areas. The heart, which is where the damage is, is referring pain to these other areas through the nervous system. To understand referred pain (sclerotome patterns), we need to visit Embryology, which is the science of development of a human during the embryonic stage. This science teaches us that the original nervous system buds out like branches of a tree. In many cases, the same nerve source will supply several different areas of our body. When pain, or damage occurs in one of the areas, by the time the Thalamus in the brain receives this information, the specific location may be distorted. Therefore, the pain normally felt in this instance is a dull ache. The source of your headache may actually be coming from your neck. A review of embryology indicates one way this can take place. The head is formed from the first and second embryonic cervical segments (the mandible from the third). [1] Therefore, the upper cervical joints (neck) can be a cause of your headaches.

Is your headache coming from your neck? Have you recently or ever damaged your neck? Neck pain and headaches are the cardinal features of whiplash. [2] 88% of patients who complained of neck pain also complained of headaches. 39.6% of those injured in a rear-end auto accident have chronic neck pain even after seven years. [3]

The nervous system will answer your question. The Trigeminal Nerve supplies the sides of your head and face. This nerve divides into three branches.

1.   Opthalmic Branch – supplies the front top of the head, temporal (side of the head), down to the nose.
2.   Maxillary Branch – Supplies the upper jaw to the upper lip.
3.   Mandibular Branch. Supplies the lower jaw. [Figure 23]

If pain is located in this area, the Trigeminal nerve must be involved. Please note in figure 21 where this nerve originates from, the Trigeminal Nucleus. This is an area located in the lower portion of your brain stem. Many understood the brainstem was located between the brain and cervical vertebra. The brain stem actually extends down in your spinal canal as low as your second or third bone in your neck. This group of grey matter has been termed the spinal fifth tract of the medulla by Seletz, [4] the Trigemino cervical nucleus of Bogduk, [5] and the Trigeminal spinal tract by Kneeft. [6] The location of the Trigeminal Nucleus is extremely important to understand. This nucleus not only receives input from the head and face, but it also receives nociceptive (pain) afferents from the sensory nerves of C1, C2, and C3. The top 3 spinal segments of your neck.

These nerves from the head, face, and top three spinal nerves travel together to the pain control center of your brain, the Thalamus. This information is difficult to decipher where the actual source of the pain is coming from. This leads to referred pain (sclerotome) to other areas not involved. Therefore, a headache felt in your head, face could actually be coming from your upper neck (most common headache).

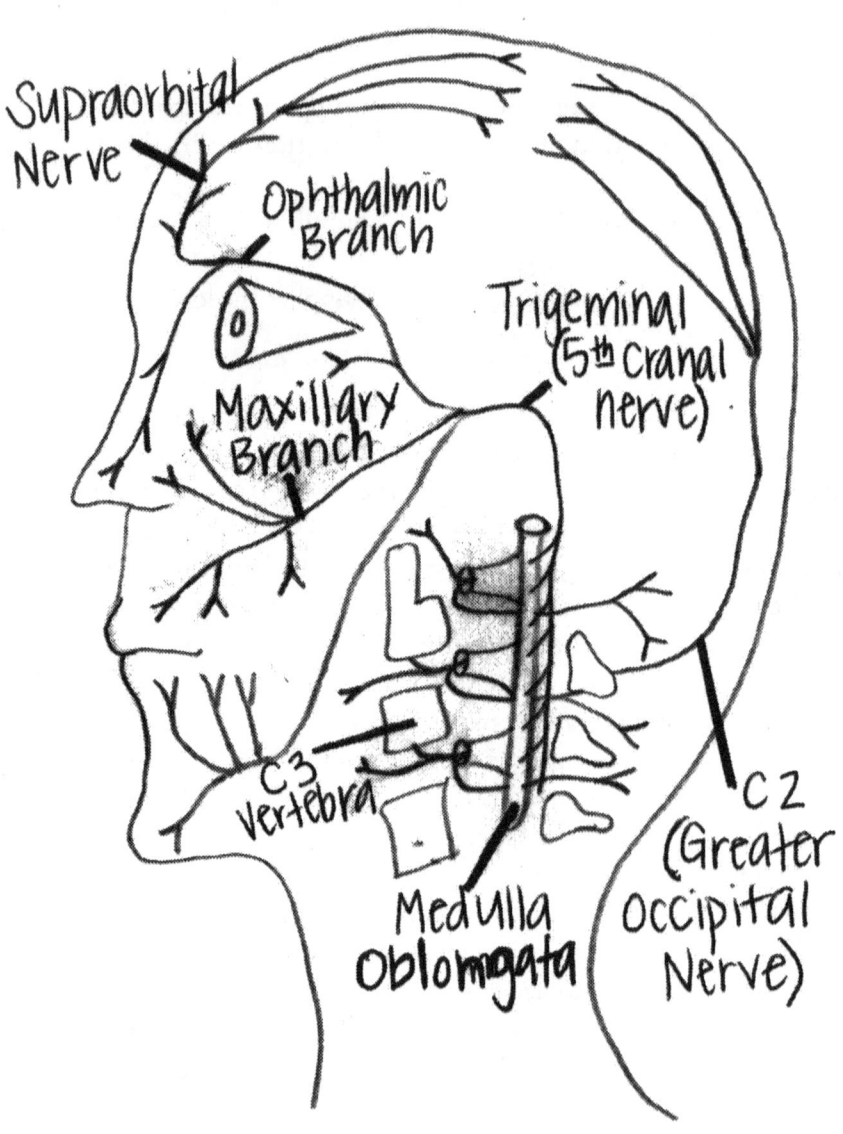

FIGURE 23

The neck has many pain sensitive structures that can cause a headache. Kreeft notes several examples – apophyseal joints (facet joints), synovial joints of the occipitoatlantial and atlantoaxial junctions, the annulas fibrosus of the intervertebral discs, spinal column ligaments, vertebral body periosteum, the cervical muscles and their attachments, cervical nerve roots, and the vertebral arteries. Trauma to these structures could refer pain to the Trigeminal Nucleus as low as C2-C4.

Seletz notes the most common area is C2 causing a headache. Rotation of the neck mostly occurs at C1/C2. There is a total of 40 degrees of rotation in one direction. The first 30 degrees of rotation occurs at C1/C2, followed by the lower cervical articulations, from above down below. Damage to the Alar ligament will cause hyper mobility in this area will lead to stretching of the tissue, leading to headaches. Damage to the Alar ligament most commonly occurs with rotation of the neck with flexion/extension, as in a patient turning, looking out the side window during a rear-end collision. This ligament is primary collagen and only stretches 10-15% before tearing. [Figure 24]

Also, if you will recall in chapter 6, we discussed where the first three nerves refer pain to the back and side of the head.

C1 – sub-occipital muscles (under the back of your skull).
C2 – A) Greater occipital nerve – (the back of your head).
      B)   lateral branch – above mastoid process and behind your ear.
      C)   Intermediate branch – communicates with the terminal branches of the supra orbital nerve.
C3 – Third occipital nerve – skin over the nostral end of the neck and occiput. [Figure 25]

The source of your headache could be coming from your neck. The intensity of your headaches, as well as frequency and duration may be controlled by you, more than you think. Review "Headache Triggers" in Chapter XI: "Treatment Considerations," for possible help.

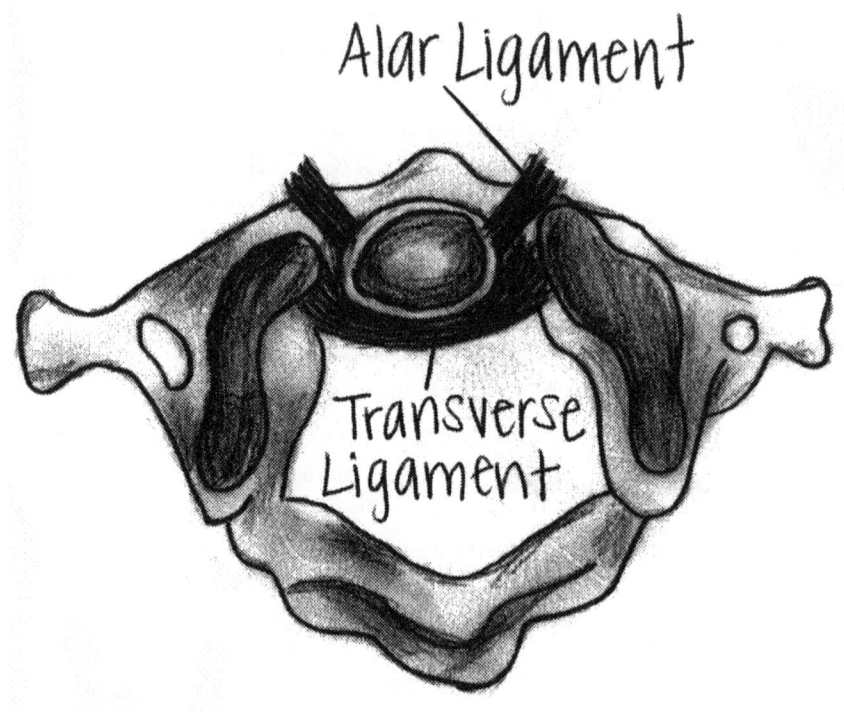

FIGURE 24

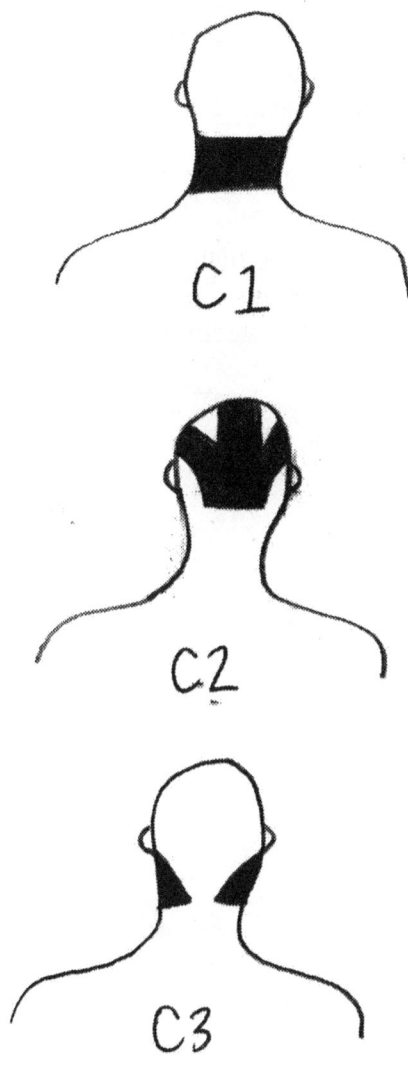

C1

C2

C3

FIGURE 25

(Endnotes)

[1] Injury to the Cervical Spine as a Cause of Headache. LesterS. Blumenthal, MD. Post Graduate Medicine. Sept. 1974. Vol. 56 No. 3

[2] The Evidence for an Organic Etiology. Arch Neurol, Vol. 57 No. 4 April 2000, 590-91.

[3] Chronic Cervical Zygopophyseal Joint Pain after Whiplash. Spine 1996; 21: 1737-1744 (August).

[4] Seletz, Emil, M.D. Whiplash Injuries, J.A.M.A., Nov 29, 1958 pp.1750-1755.

[5] Bogduk, N., Ph. D., The Anatomical Basis for Cervicogenic Headache. JMPT, Jan. 1992, pp. 67-70

[6] Kreept, J. Headache Following Whiplash, in Spine: State of the Art Reviews: Cervical Flexion – Extension/Whiplash Injuries, Sept. 1993 p. 395

CHAPTER X

BLURRED VISION

The most common complaint during consultation is "when I pick up the newspaper or a book and first try to read it, everything appears blurry. But once I hold the newspaper very still and I concentrate on one word at a time, I can read it." Sounds too familiar.

In order to see objects in your life, the eyeballs must be able to move around in your eye sockets to fix the focus in your eyes, on what you are looking at. You have several muscles surrounding the eye to move it all around. [Figure 26] These muscles are controlled by cranial nerves coming from your brain stem. The nucleus (control center) of these cranial nerves originate in the brain stem. These control centers decipher the information from sensory nerves going to them, and in direct response from that sensory input, control the eyeballs with their motor (muscle) control. This is a very important concept you need to understand before you read any further. The nervous system in your body has control centers located in different areas to control certain functions in your body. This is necessary for you to live and exist. These control centers rely on receiving information from sensory nerves going into them, and respond to these signals with motor or hormonal control with nerves going out of the control centers. The sensory input, or information control centers receive are from many sources in your body.

For instance, let us focus on the control center for one eye muscle, the Lateral Rectus. This muscle is on the outside of the eye balls, and specifically move the eye laterally, to the outside of your socket. The specific cranial nerve controlling the Lateral Rectus muscle is called Abducens. This cranial nerve comes from the middle of your brain stem. [Figure 27] This nucleus does not decide to move the eye laterally,

73

by stimulating the Lateral Rectus muscle by itself. The control center receives information from other sensory nerves outside of the brain stem to help coordinate the degree and speed of outward movement necessary at that instant. If the information the control center receives is not correct or the information is altered for some reason, the control center reacts as if this information was the Gospel Truth. If a nerve going to the Abducens control center is irritated and sending information, which is not accurate due to this irritation, then the lateral rectus muscle would be stimulated to move the eye at an inappropriate time, leading to blurred vision. Let us look a little further into this area to understand a little better if this possibly could be your problem.

In order for humans to see objects, the muscles of the eyes position the eyes to focus on the particular target at that time. Two mechanisms, which are responsible for this is known as Saccade and Smooth Pursuit.

Dorland's Medical Dictionary states "Saccade – The series of involuntary, abrupt, rapid, small movements or jerks of both eyes simultaneously in changing the point of fixation." Saccade allows the eyes to focus on an object rapidly in the periphery. This movement is extremely fast, even up to 900 degrees per second. This reaction is a very important protective device in case of an object moving fast toward you.

Smooth Pursuit's function is to coordinate the eyes focusing on a moving target. In order for this to occur, smooth pursuit must actually calculate how fast the target is moving to allow clear vision of the target. Any time you are watching a moving object, for instance a baseball thrown to you, you are utilizing your smooth pursuit. The control center of this phenomenon is located in the lower part of your brain stem (medulla oblongata), and is called the Vestibular Nucleus. (Please note the location of this control center). [Figure 28] The vestibular nucleus must have input from other sources to maintain coordinated smooth pursuit. The following is a simplified series of events taking place at the same time for this coordinated movement.

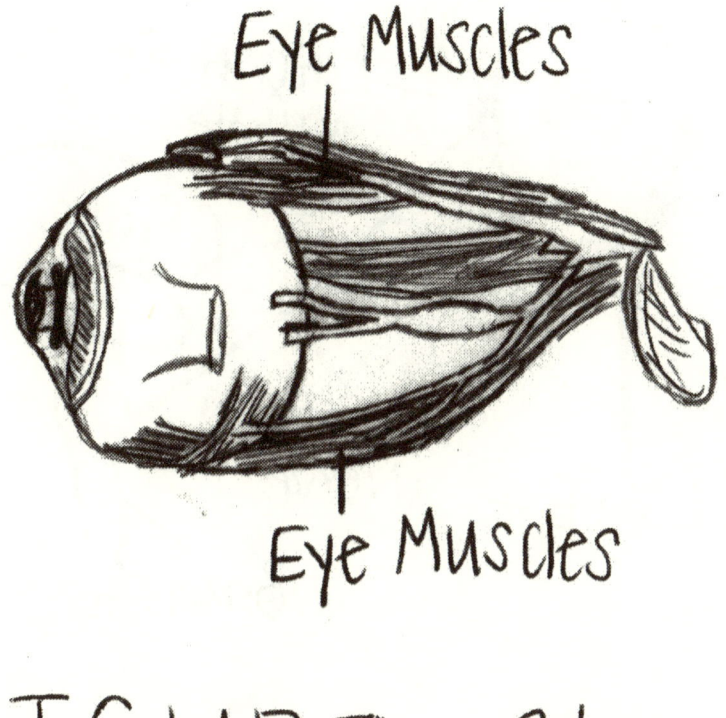

FIGURE 26

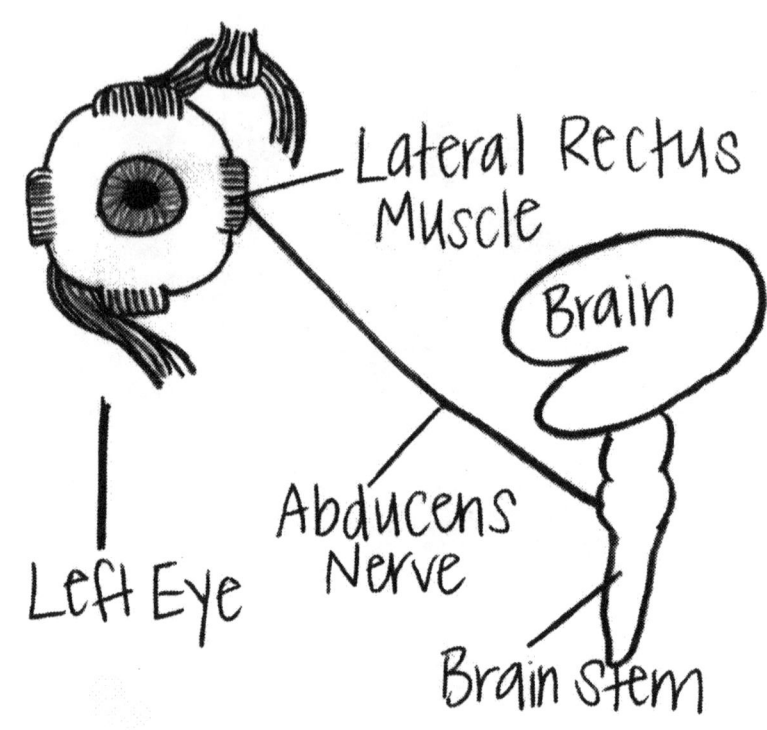

Lateral Rectus Muscle

Brain

Left Eye

Abducens Nerve

Brain Stem

FIGURE 27

The Vestibular Nucleus:

1. Receives information from the Cerebellus (Flocculus and Vermis) Note: The Flocculus and Vermis relay the information necessary to determine the velocity of the target being followed. These areas also receive information from the outer portion of the brain (cerebral cortex).
2. Relays information to the Abducens Nucleus located in the brain stem above. Note: The Abducens Nucleus controls the lateral eye muscles (Lateral Rectus).
3. Relays information to the Oculomotor Nuclei located in the brain stem above. Note: Oculomotor Nucleus – controls other eye muscles.

This system must have outside information relayed to it necessary for coordinated eye movement to maintain clear vision. If there is a problem in any of the above areas, for instance a disruption or irritated nerves, it would prevent someone from making adequate smooth pursuit eye movements. Instead, they would follow a moving target by utilizing a combination of altered or defective smooth pursuit movements and small saccades (fast, jerky movements). [1]

The combination of eye movements trying to focus on an object would explain blurred vision on any, even slightly moving object. If you keep the object, newspaper, etc., very still and not move your head, focusing becomes possible with clear vision.

[Physicians should note: Patients with brainstem or cerebellar lesions cannot pursue targets moving toward the side of the lesion.]

In Sweden, a study was performed on 27 patients, two years after whiplash injury. Their symptoms included neck pain, headaches, vertigo, nausea, blurring of vision, dysacusis (hearing impairment), fullness of the ear, and various emotional and cognitive disturbances. They were compared to a control group, subjects without a history of whiplash injury.

Two tests utilized:
1. Kinesthetic Sensibility Test:
   a. All subjects had vision occluded by goggles
   b. A laser pointer was fixed to a helmet on their head.

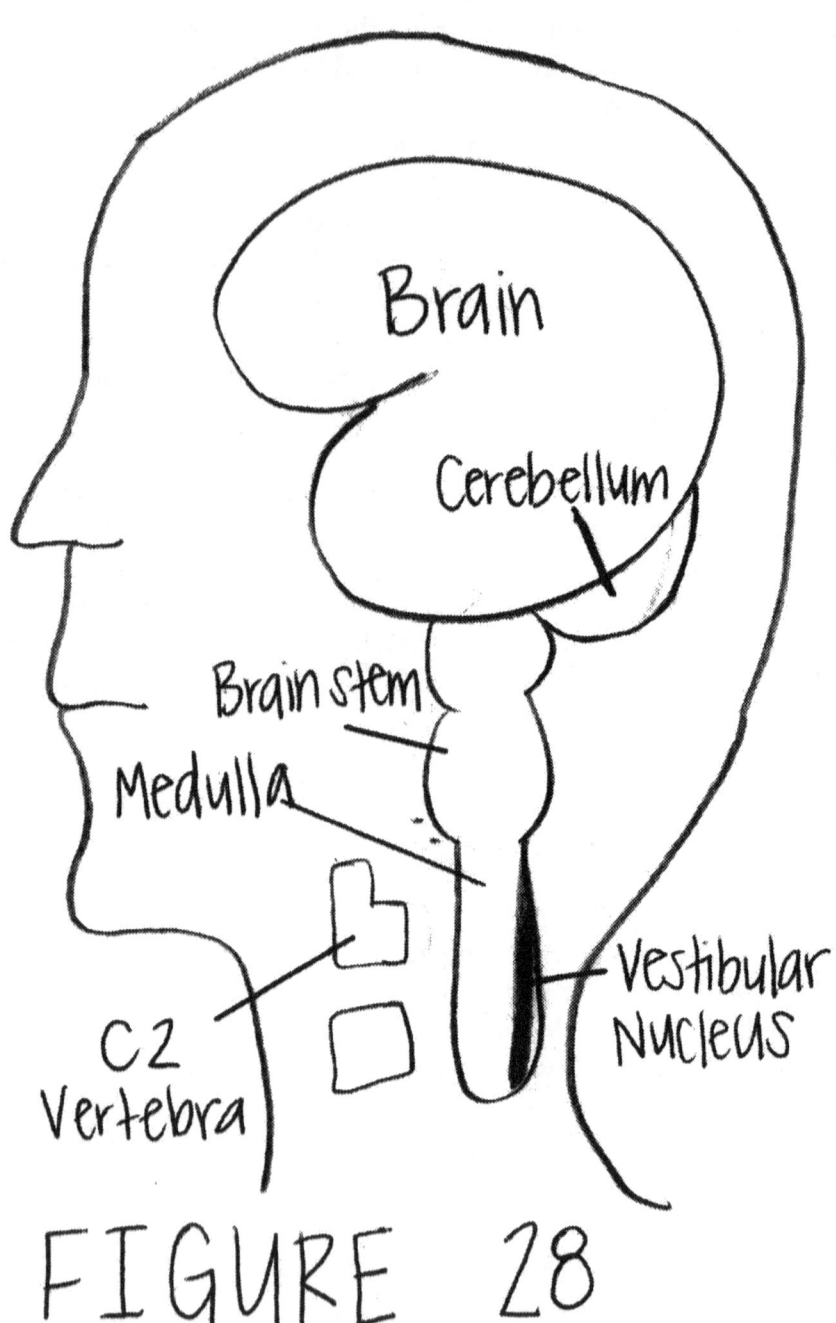

Brain

Cerebellum

Brain stem

Medulla

Vestibular Nucleus

C2 Vertebra

FIGURE 28

      c. They were instructed to concentrate on a target position, follow by maximally rotating their head to the left, for 21 seconds – then trying to locate the initial focused area.

      d. The relocation accuracy was measured in centimeters from the center of the initial target

      e. 10 trials

      f. Repeated for right rotation.

      g. 27 patients were compared to 39 healthy subjects (24 women, 15 men).

2. Oculomotor Test

      a. Side to side (horizontal) eye movement tests were recorded by a computer.

      b. Test performed on all 26 patients two years after whiplash injury.

      c. They were compared to 25 healthy subjects.

Discussion

"Our study was concerned with the capacity of patients with whiplash injury to relocate the head in space after an active displacement by moving the head away from a reference position. Repositioning dysfunction was present in 62% of subjects with whiplash trauma two years after the trauma. Patients with whiplash injury return the head to the reference position with significantly less accuracy than healthy subjects.

"These results suggest that restriction of cervical movement and changes in the quality of proprioceptive information from the cervical spine region affect voluntary eye movement."

"No correlations between age and oculomotor and kinesthetic sensibility were observed for the control group." "For whiplash subjects age and sex seem to correlate with cervical kinesthetic performances and with oculomotor functions. This fact could indicate that elderly people and women are more vulnerable to injuries affecting the proprioceptive systems."

Conclusion

"Proprioceptive dysfunction might be one of the most important factors for understanding the morbidity after a non-contact whiplash trauma to the neck."

Discussion

These results suggest that damage to the mechano-receptors and altered neck motion following a whiplash injury changes the quality of proprioceptive input from the cervical spine affecting eye movements. There by concluding, Oculomotor dysfunction after whiplash injuries might be related to disturbances related to the input from the neck. References:[2.]

(Endnotes)

[1.] SACCADE AND SMOOTH PURSUIT.   Kandel, Schantz, Jessel. Principles of Neural Science, 2000

[2.] "Cervicocephalic Kinesthetic Sensibility, Active Range of Motion, and Oculomotor Function in Patients with Whiplash Injury." Arch Phys. Med. Rehabil 79(9): 1089-94. Heikkila, H.V. and B.-1. Wenngren (1998)

CHAPTER XI

DIZZINESS/LOSS OF COORDINATION

Stedman's Medical Dictionary defines:

dizziness – Imprecise term commonly used to describe various symptoms such as faintness, giddiness, imbalance, light-headedness, unsteadiness, or vertigo.

Coordination – The harmonious working together of several muscles or muscle groups in the execution of complicated movements.

Following trauma to the cervical spine, or even slow, chronic pathologies leading to decreased neck motions, leads to dizziness and loss of coordination. The nerves responsible for this reaction are known as mechano-receptors. Dorland's Medical Dictionary defines mechanoreceptors – A receptor that is excited by mechanical pressure or distortions, as those responding to sound, touch, and muscular contractions. Specific types are variously called corpuscles, nerve endings, and receptors.

Dr. Barry Wyke, Director of the Neurological Unit of the Royal College of Surgeons in England, tells us All synovial joints of the body, without exception, are provided with a distinct set of receptors. These sensory nerves that relay information to the brain, controls our coordination more than we realize.

There are four types of these mechano-receptors.

Type I – Corpuscles
   – located in fibrous capsule at junction of synovial tissue
   – has low threshold if tension
   – continuous firing persists.
   – biggest contribution in accuracy of control.

<u>Type 2</u> – Corpuscles at synovial joints/at junction of fibrous
corpuscles
- low threshold
- quick firing
- short
- only at initial movement
- always motor response.

<u>Type 3</u> – Corpuscles in ligaments
- high threshold
- continuous firing if tension remains high
- located at attachments
- do not fire with minor or moderate tension
- very flat at surface of ligaments
- clustered at attachment at both ends
- free nerve endings in myelinated throughout the entire ligament.

When the joint is immobile – tonic static discharge from Type 1 receptor. When stretch joints, Type 1 is augmented and returned to normal discharge when at resting position. Type 2 receptors emit only a very brief at change or tension. They don't fire during immobilization.

Type 1 receptors are relayed throughout the central nervous system, eventually to the paracentral and parietal regions of the cerebral cortex, where they make major contribution to postural sensation (one's conscious awareness of the static position of one's joints) and to kinesthesis (one's conscious assessment of the direction, velocity, and amplitude of joint movement) generated actively or passively.

Dr. Wyke continues to tell us if you take a normal subject anesthetize the joint capsule – their capacity to recognize accurately the static position of that joint with the eyes closed and their capacity to the amplitude and velocity of an imposed joint movement is very grossly impaired, but not completely abolished. This person's accuracy of kinesthesis would also be grossly impaired. If mechano-receptors are destroyed, as in Rheumatoid or Osteo Arthritis, or destroyed by direct joint trauma (auto-accident), then all such patients show impairment of postural sensation and of kinesthesis related to the affected joint.

If you immobilize a joint (cervical collar), the corpuscular mechano-receptors begin to disappear, and after a period of six weeks- two months, there are no mechano-receptors left in any of the joint capsules.

Partial loss of the normal mechano-receptor input from receptors in a joint capsule has profound consequences for kinesthetic reflex control.

The cervical spine contains mostly type I-III proprioceptive mechanoreceptors. The lumbar spine contains mostly Type IV nociceptive (pain) mechano-receptors.

The most important regulator of balance are from the mechano-receptors in the cervical spine. Far more input than from the vestibular system. In normal cervical spine mechano-receptors, it can compensate totally for an absolute vestibular deficit. No disturbance of posture, gait, and conscious awareness of balance.

Dr. Wyke continues "If altered/deficient cervical mechano-receptors- total compensation of vestibular system is impossible. Discharges from the cervical mechano-receptors, particularly those from the upper 4, are transmitted cephalad to the motor neuron pools of the eye muscles, jaw muscles, and to the tongue musculature. This explains why after events such as whiplash, the patients show disturbance of eye movements (nystagmus), disturbance of speech articulation, and sometimes problems while chewing, and disturbance of balance, posture, and gait. This syndrome is usually blamed on vestibular damage or to inadequate blood flow in the basiler artery."

Type I receptors are primarily responsible for postural and Kinesthetic sensation of head and neck. (One's conscious awareness of movement of head or neck.) Influence on one facet joint affects not only bilateral, but also to the motor neuron pools of all the muscles, including the limb muscles.

Very interesting research –

Objective – To evaluate impairment of proprioception quantitatively in patients with cervical myelopathy.

Methods – The authors evaluated knee proprioception in 54 cervical myelopathy patients and compared results with those of 54 age-matched healthy volunteers. Knee proprioception was assessed by joint position sense, represented by the emor angles when patients reproduced pre-determined angles of knee flexion.

Discussion

Sensory information concerning proprioception is mediated by specialized nerve endings, called mechanoreceptors, which are located in the joint capsules, ligaments, muscles, tendons, and skin. The receptors transduce the mechanical stimulus energy of joints into the electrical energy of a nerve action potential. These neural impulses travel in the posterior columns of the spinal cord toward the cerebral cortex. Thus, disorders only where in these neural pathways can cause proprioceptive deterioration.

In conclusion, the results of the present study demonstrate impairment of knee position sense in patients with cervical myelopathy. It is known that proprioception plays an important role in smooth and coordinated activation of the limbs. Therefore, the functional status in the lower extremities of patients with cervical myelopathy is affected by impairment of proprioception. [1.]

Let us review the previous material. There are nerves (mechano-receptors)in your neck that play a tremendous part in controlling your balance. These nerves respond and relay information to the balance control centers as your neck joints move. Trauma can damage these nerves, as well as restricting neck motion. If this is true, would you expect someone's balance to decrease if we restricted their neck movements? There was actual research to study the "Halo Vest Effect on Balance." Note: A Halo Vest is commonly used to maximally restrict patients from any neck motions.

OBJECTIVE: To determine the effect of a halo vest, a cervical orthesis, on clinically relevant balance parameters.

DESIGN: Subjects performed unipedal stance (with eyes open and closed, on both firm and soft surfaces) and functional reach, with and without the application of a halo vest.

Discussion

The major finding of this study was that healthy young subjects demonstrated a decrease in both unipedal stance time and functional reach with a halo vest compared to without one. Although we found a clear impairment in balance with the acute use of a halo vest, our study may underestimate the real impact of a halo vest on a postural stability. Given that a halo vest is usually worn for three to four months, the impact on balance may be much greater in clinical practice. Furthermore, many patients who require a halo vest may have a period of bed rest, a myelopathy, or other neurological or orthopedic trauma that will impair balance further. Therefore, the decrement in balance we found in healthy subjects would likely be amplified in a typical patient population.

Cervical muscle proprioception has been found to influence eye movement and balance. Stabilizing the neck would prevent cervical muscle motion and likely lessen the efficiency of the involved proprioceptors, while stabilizing the head may prevent optimal positioning of the vestibular apparatus. Given the likely mechanisms of this impairment and findings from previous research, it is likely that the impairment would be greater in older or injured patients who are required to wear a halo vest for a period of months. [2.]

The conclusion is simple. Damage to your neck mechanoreceptors, or restricted neck motions could lead to loss of balance, dizziness, blurred vision, or loss of coordination.

(Endnotes)

1. Hiroyuki Takoyoma, MC, Hirostugu Muratsu, M.D., Minoru Doita, M.D., Toshihiko Haroda, M.D., Shini
2. James K. Richardson, M.D., Alahn D. Marr Ross, M.D., Barth Riley, PH.D. Robert L. Rhodes, MPA, Co. Halo Vest Effect on Balance. Arch Phys Med Rehabil Vol 81, March 2000, pp. 255-257.

Chapter XII

Treatment Considerations

This chapter is not designed to reveal a recipe for treatment. A physician should always be consulted. This information is exactly what the title suggests, treatment considerations. Referring back to Proverbs 4:7, "Yet in all thy getting, get <u>understanding</u>. Patients are much more intelligent today, researching on the computer their diagnosis. I am only suggesting you continue your inquisitive nature past your diagnosis, and understand your treatment.

Let us keep this chapter simple. Your symptoms are a result of aberrant, altered function somewhere in your body. Something is not working right. The key to treatment is finding the specific problem, not only subsiding the symptoms. Once we find the specific problem, our goal should be to assist the body in restoring normal function, when possible. For example, if you have a splinter in your finger, the body will respond with inflammation at the site and the swelling and chemicals in the area will cause pain. Pain medication will help your symptoms, but PLEASE will someone pull out the splinter? Fix the problem, and the annoying symptoms will go away.

The majority of you have received trauma to your neck, as in an automobile accident. Let us try and understand what takes place on a cellular level. In chapter IV, figure 13 revealed how ligaments are damaged in your neck during an automobile accident. The ligament tissue cells are actually torn. When a cell is torn, a response occurs immediately to begin the healing process.

The first step is known as the inflammation process. This step is vital for not only initial treatment, but also it attracts the cells necessary to restore normal ligament tissue/function. Inflammation is the dynamic process, which occurs when these damaged ligament cells release chemicals in the surrounding tissue, causing a reaction.

INFLAMMATION – A protective tissue response to injury or destruction of tissues, which serves to destroy, dilute, or wall off both the injurious agent and the injured tissues. The classical signs of acute inflammation are pain , heat, redness, swelling, and loss of function. – Dorland's Medical Dictionary.

As we discuss the steps of the inflammation process, keep in mind these steps are not simply step 1, step 2, etc. These processes overlap each other, and are taking place at the same time, on occasions. When a cell is damaged, it releases a chemical, Histamine, to increase the permeability of the local blood vessels. This increases the circulation to the local area to bring and take away substances needed for healing the local damaged tissue. This increase in circulation appears red on the surface of the body.

The damaged cells of the body need to be taken away by the white blood cells. The white blood cells are wandering along in the blood vessels and in the tissue. They are negatively charged as well as the blood vessel wall. This wall repels the white blood cells, keeping the cells moving in the middle of the blood vessel (axial stream). In inflammation, this vessel lining changes to a positive charge. This attracts the needed white blood cells. Then a process occurs, known as DIAPEDESIS – the movement of white blood cells and other cells out of small arterioles, venules, and capillaries, as part of the inflammatory response (TABER'S MEDICAL DICTIONARY). These cells move through the gaps between cells in the vessel walls. The red blood cells are also negatively charged, and a number of them may follow the white blood cells. The blood plasma also follows the solid cells into the damaged tissue area. This reaction is responsible for most of the localized swelling of the damaged area. This slows the flow of the blood stream in these local vessels. This can lead to damaging congestion.

Therefore, initially, the first treatment consideration should be the use of ice, not heat. In order to limit the damaging effects of the initial swelling, ice placed on the affected area will result in the blood vessels to constrict, get smaller in diameter. This vaso-constriction leads to decreased swelling, congestion, hemorrhage, and temperature. Ice therapy will decrease the severity of local cellular damage by restricting hemorrhage and edema.

When placing an ice pack on damaged tissue, the complete area should be covered. Always place a cloth between the ice source and the skin to prevent any damage to the skin. Ice normally leads to four different sensations. First, it will naturally feel cold, followed second by a burning sensation. The third sensation will be an ache. This ache sensation is normally the shortest sensation. Finally, the fourth sensation is a numb, anesthetic sensation.

A word of caution using ice. The initial effects of ice will cause the blood vessels to constrict, decreasing the swelling. However, if you ice the damaged area too long (the body tissue's core temperature gets too cold), the body will react to our opposite desire. Vascular dilation will occur (blood vessels expanding), allowing blood to warm the area back towards normal. The phenomenon will lead to even more congestion than if we never used ice. Therefore, to prevent the damaged tissue from becoming too cold, ice packs should be applied at intervals. For instance, on a thick large neck, ice can be applied 30 minutes on, 30 minutes off, then back on for 30 minutes. A smaller, less dense area, such as a finger, apply ice packs 15 minutes on, 15 minutes off, and 15 minutes back on. This process could be repeated several times a day.

The next treatment consideration – Should I wear a neck brace? Referring back to figure 3 in chapter 2. If the damage to your neck could compromise your spinal cord, you should have your neck immobilized. This is not the usual, however.

Before a neck brace is used, let us first review our treatment goal, to help restore normal function. In an automobile accident, the ligaments are stressed quickly beyond their limits, and intrinsic tears occur throughout the ligament (figure 13). These tears diminish the strength, and "rubber band" stretchiness of the ligaments allowing the specific bones they attach to, to move extra. Our goal should be aimed at allowing the body to fill the damaged torn areas with the normal ligament tissue. It shouldn't be hard to understand if this damaged area is replaced with hardened scar tissue, the ligament will not return to its original rubber band self. This would allow the bones to continue to move extra. If you wear a cervical collar (immobilize), this will lead to scar tissue formation, instead of normal collagen ligament tissue. Also to consider, when you stop moving a joint of the body, the involved muscles will atrophy and weaken. Immobilization may lead to decreased recovery with long term rehabilitative outcomes.

The next key phase of the inflammation process is known as the proliferative phase. This phase includes a vital cell proliferation, known as fibroblasts.

Fibroblasts – Any cell or corpuscle from which connective tissue is developed; it produces collagen, elastin, and reticular protein fibers. "Taber's Medical Dictionary"

In the proliferation phase, inflammatory cells eliminate the damaged tissue cells by phagocytosis. We need normal collagen fiber filling in the torn gaps in the ligament tissue. The fibroblasts markedly elevate collagen production. This initial collagen filling these gaps are weaker collagen. Later, ideally this weak collagen will mature from type 3 to type I, normal, mature, tough and stretchy, original collagen.

Key Question: Can we influence the damaged ligament to return closer to normal, original Type I collagen tissue?

The answer begins with passive motion. What is passive motion?

No motion = Neck brace (immobilization)

Active motion = Your neck is moved by using your muscles.

Passive Motion = Occurs when the joints in your neck are mobilized by submission to another source of energy.

For instance, hold your index finger with your other hand. Now, move your index finger around, only actively using your other hand, while relaxing your index finger. This is passive motion. Movement without localized muscle activity. Now that you basically understand passive motion, let us review research on this subject.

STUDY #1

Hypothesis: Continuous passive motion of a synovial joint would have a beneficial biological effect on the healing of full-thickness defects in articular cartilage.

Experimental Model: Using an electrical dental drill, full thickness defects, one millimeter in diameter, were made in the articular cartilage and subchondral bone to a standard depth four millimeters of the knees of 120 adolescent rabbits and 27 adult rabbits.

Group1 – After drilling hole – knees were casted (immobilized)
Group 2 - After drilling hole – placed rabbits in a large cage and did not restrict activity.

Group 3 - After drilling hole, continuous passive motion of knees by placing the joint in a machine flexing and extending the knee automatically.

NATURE OF REPARATIVE TISSUE
(what tissue filled the holes in the knee?)

Adolescent Group

Group 1 – (cast immobilization)
- o   After three weeks – 85% scar tissue
- o   After ten weeks – all but two of the thirty defects – the holes were covered by fibrous tissue, adhesive (scar tissue)

Group 2 – (Active Motion)
- o   After three weeks – 75% scar tissue
- o   After four weeks – 80% of the defects filled with scar tissue

Group 3 – (Passive Motion)
- o   After three weeks – cells replacing drilled holes in 52% were normal chondrocyte cells.

ADULT GROUP

Group 1 – (Cast Immobilization)
- o   After three weeks – 86% scar tissue

Group2 – (Active Motion)
- o   After 3 weeks – 81% scar tissue

Group 3 – (Passive Motion)
o   After 3 weeks – 31% scar tissue

Conclusion – Continuous passive motion stimulates much more rapid and more complete healing of full thickness defects in the articular cartilage of rabbits' knees than does either immobilization or intermittent active motion. [1.]

STUDY #2

The purpose of this study is to compare passive motion vs. mobilization. The adult dog was chosen because of similarities in the flex – or apparatus of humans and dogs, and because of the necessity of having animals pre-trained for a full mobilization and exercise program.

Using 30 adult Mongrel dogs, the left second and fourth tendons of the toes were cut. The cut tendons were then sutured back together and all were initially immobilized with a cast.
The dogs were divided into six groups.

Group 1 – three weeks of immobilization

Group 2 – six weeks of immobilization

Group 3 – three weeks of immobilization, three weeks of full weight bearing mobilization

Group 4 – three weeks of immobilization, three weeks of partial mobilization (wrist 90 degrees)

Group 5 – three weeks of immobilization, six weeks of partial mobilization (three weeks wrist 90 degrees/ three weeks 45 degrees)

Group 6 – three weeks of immobilization, nine weeks of partial mobilization (three weeks at 45 degrees/three weeks at neutral).

Note: To achieve passive mobilization the wrist and toes were fully flexed and extended to their limits, five minutes daily.

Results

Group 1 - blood vessels located only at the level of reconnected tendon when studied by cross-section.

Group 2 – After six weeks of immobilization, decrease of blood supply as compared to group 1. No blood vessels were found within the tendon more than 2 mm. From the cut area.

Group 3 – All tendons ruptured prior to the study.

Group 4 – No moderate increase of blood vessels compared with group 2. The cross section study revealed an increase of blood vessels in the previous cut tendons.

Group 5 – A reduction of blood vessels in peritendinous compared to group 4. The vessels were more oblique and longitudinal in orientation and of equal density in zones II, III, and IV

Group 6 – The vessels were less dense and more longitudinally oriented than in group 5. The more distal zones were most vascular. The vascularity of these tendons regained some of the normal characteristics of normal tendons.

Conclusion – A gradually increasing range of passive motion was associated with the blood vessels returning back to normal. [2.]

Therefore, an important treatment consideration is controlled PASSIVE MOTION. Recall our primary goal is to assist the body in returning the tissue back to the original Type I collagen fibers. (Refer to Figure 6). We would like to guard against scar tissue formation and to prevent excess formation of the weaker type III collagen that can contribute to chronic elongation of the ligament. Shortly after the injury, the collagen tissue starts to mature. During this phase, controlled passive motion on the damaged ligament will promote proper collagen fiber orientation. The ideal controlled passive motion should bring a joint (vertebrae) through their normal range of motion, through their normal axis of rotation.

The type I collagen consists of three procollagen chains associated at one end by means of their extension peptides, intertwining as cross-links are formed- to give the triple Helix of the procollagen molecule. The direction of the fiber formation appears to be dependent on the stresses acting on the tissue.

Controlled muscle stretching and joint movement enhance new collagen fiber orientation parallel to the stress lines of the normal collagen fibers. The maturation of tendon and ligament tissue may take as long as six to twelve months. [3.] Early mobilization is the best method to avoid joint contracture and its harmful consequences on articular cartilage. The technique also serves to maintain and return joint proprioception, which, in turn, may be important in preventing re-injury and in hastening recovery to full fitness. Therefore, the technique can be recommended as the method of choice for acute – soft tissue injury. [3.]

Atrophy, shrinking of the muscles, should be avoided when possible. Atrophied, weakened muscles will allow local joint motion to be altered. Hopefully we now understand altered joint motion will stimulate the local proprioceptive fibers, leading to altered function. The best method for preventing disuse atrophy is usage. A controlled rehab program including isometric/isotonic/muscle stretching exercises should be considered to help restore normal joint motion, especially if the local ligaments are damaged. Active motion will also help with pain control. Recall active motion is using your own muscles to move your joints. The sensation of pain is carried to your brain (thalamus) by small diameter afferents (nerves). Large diameter afferents are nerves that carry the impulses from our mechano-receptors. Recall mechano-receptors are located in our joints and muscle spindles, which carry the activity of movement to the brain. "The perception of pain is dependant upon the balance of activity between large diameter and small diameter afferents." Increasing the firing of large diameter fibers (mechano-receptors) diminish the small diameter fibers (pain).

This explains how we can diminish our pain during continued active movement. The active motion should not be continued however, where ligament damage is located. The decrease of pain may occur initially, however, extra motion will irritate the local damaged area, creating an inflammatory response. When the activity diminishes, the small diameter afferents dominate, causing pain. This explains the typical whiplash patient. Their pain cycle is up and down like a roller coaster. They will have a good day without much pain, They will unknowingly actively move their head around more due to lack of pain. During this time of active movement, they are firing their large diameter nerve fiber (mechano-receptors) which diminish the pain even more. However, during this movement they irritated the tissue, which is moving extra, due to damaged ligaments. This will initiate an inflammatory response, which will cause localized swelling over night. The following morning, they are in pain again, and can't even think about moving their head the wrong way due to too much pain. Sound too familiar?

If you are victimized with HEADACHES, treating your damaged ligaments may not be the only cause of your problem. Headache TRIGGERS must be understood and considered when dealing with headaches. Let us keep this discussion as simple as possible. Before your pain nerves will fire, they must reach a threshold of stimuli to activate pain. This stimuli could be of many sources. For instance, let us say before a pain nerve fiber will fire, and give you the sensation of pain, this nerve must receive a total of 100 stimuli. The ligaments in your neck are damaged, allowing extra movement between C1 and C2 vertebra. This will cause the pain nerve to reach 90 stimuli, which is not quite 100. You drink a cold, tall glass of milk, not realizing you're lactose intolerant (your body cannot break down the sugar in the milk), and this gives the pain nerve seven stimuli. Nerves will summate (add) their stimuli. This is a total of 97. On top of all this, you have to give a speech at your employment to a group of over 200 people. This added stress will add 15 stimuli. The total of 112 stimuli will fire the pain nerve, and you now have a headache. Increasing triggers will lead to headaches increasing in intensity, frequency, and duration. Do you have any headache triggers? They may include:

Stress	Hunger or low blood sugar
Alcohol or Caffeine	A change in sleep patterns
Hormonal Changes	A change in the weather
Wheat	Polluted air
Chocolate	Stuffy rooms
Scents, odors (perfumes)	Smoke
Nuts	Cheese Products
Monosodium Glutamate	Vinegar
Bright Lights	Yeast
Cleaning Products	Aspartame (Nutra Sweet)
Physical Exertion	Possibly certain fruits and juices
	Tennis, Biking, etc.

The list is unending! The trick is to determine your specific triggers. A simple technique is to start keeping a headache diary. It is easy, extremely informative, and only takes a few minutes. Whenever you have a headache log the date (for frequency), the time it occurred (duration), and how severe the headache was (intensity – scale 1-10, where 1 is a very light headache and 10 is a suicidal headache). If someone is trying to help you with your headaches, you should see a decrease of the frequency, intensity, and duration of your headaches. Possible triggers must be included. You need to include food, physical activity, beverages, possible stress or weather change, anything that could possibly add stimuli to this specific headache. I would list everything for the previous 24 hours. Yes, I know this will take a little time, but this information is priceless. In a short amount of time, you will start noticing common denominators that frequent your previous 24 hour list. By eliminating your possible triggers, you may not be able to eliminate your headaches, but you may see a dramatic decrease in the frequency, intensity, and duration of your headaches.

ANALGESIC REBOUND HEADACHES

"Analgesic agents are prescription or over-the-counter medications used to control pain including migraine and other types of headaches. When used on a daily or near daily basis, these analgesics can perpetuate the headache process. They may decrease the intensity of the pain for a few hours; however they appear to feed into the pain system in such a way that chronic headaches may result. If under these circumstances the patient does not completely stop using these analgesics, despite any other treatment undertaken, the chronic headache is likely to continue unabated." [4.]

Usually when analgesics are discontinued the headache may get worse for several days and the sufferer may experience nausea or vomiting. However, after a period of three to five days, sometimes longer, these symptoms begin to improve. For those patients willing to persevere, the headaches will gradually improve as response to more appropriate medication occurs. Most patients are able to stop the use of analgesics at home under physician supervision, but some find it difficult and may require hospitalization, as many sufferers have been using analgesics several times a day for many years." [5.]

Therefore, medications, including over-the-counter meds should be included in your headache diary. The meds, or the lack of these meds could be one of your major headache triggers.

<u>Manipulative Procedures</u>

"These therapies are broadly grouped by the fact that they require a skilled practitioner to move joints or muscles in an effort to relieve tension in the muscle and promote normal joint mechanics, mobilize fluids within soft tissues and promote normalcy or neural function and movement. These therapies include osteopathic manipulation performed by a doctor of osteopathy (D.O.), chiropractic manipulation performed by a chiropractor (D.C.) or muscle manipulation performed by physical therapists or myofascial therapists. Specific Techniques such as Rolfing, Alexander, and Feldenkrais are also types of manipulation. All of these therapies have certain nuances in how they are performed that set them apart from one another, but it is probably fair to say the skill of the practitioner is central to their success. These therapies are most likely to be useful when muscle tension is a key part of the headaches or there has been an injury to the head or spinal region, especially the neck." [5.]

Active physical rehabilitation has many benefits. The term "Active" means you are actually, physically completing the exercise. If there is a joint in the body unstable, where the two bones joined together are moving extra strengthening the surrounding muscles will help restore motion closer to normal (in some cases). Therefore, isotonic active exercises of the appropriate surrounding muscles are extremely beneficial. When you lift the weight, this causes muscle contraction. This squeezing of the muscle actively circulates the blood in the affected area. This new blood circulation brings with it fresh oxygen for cellular energy, as well as needed nutrients to help restore normal local damaged tissue. Active muscle contraction also stimulates lymphatic flow. When there is extra fluid, swelling in our tissues, our lymphatic system helps drain the extra fluid causing unnecessary congestion and pain.

The adult human disc is the largest avascular structure in the body. In adult discs, some cells may be as much as 6 to 8mm from the nearest blood supply, which resides in the osseous end plate of the adjacent vertebral bodies. The mineralized portion of the endplate is penetrated by marrow contact channels, through which capillary buds emerge. Several studies have demonstrated that the central region of the endplate is the predominant route of transport for metabolic processes of the disc. [6.]

Please recall a whiplash injury occurs in less than 150- ms. after impact. During this crucial time, compression is the result of upward thrust of the trunk while the lower cervical segments consistently exceed physiological limits of posterior rotation. This abnormal rotation around an abnormal axis of rotation causes the anterior ends of adjacent vertebral bodies to separate, resulting in disc injury.

Injuries of vertebral endplate maybe one of the pathomechanisms leading to early changes in the disc matrix and eventually to abnormal biomechanical behavior of the whole disc. [7.]

The disc degeneration has often an impact on the facet joints, which suffer loss of articular space, deformation of the facets, hypertrophic osteophytes, and finally segment instability. Destabilization and the resulting unphysiologic movements can lead to accelerated disc degeneration and may consequently lead to pain and neurological deficit. One possible approach to the management of disc disease would be to apply dynamic distraction to the disc at an early time point to increase disc height, stimulating disc diffusion, resulting in increased water content and finally leading to increased disc nutrition.

In the current study, we stimulated disc regeneration to the degenerated rabbit intervertebral disc. Dynamic mechanical distraction may play an important part in revising the effect of disc degeneration. Early intervention when disc degeneration was initiated seems to be important to maintain disc health or stimulate tissue repair. [8.]

The key to successful treatment is the understanding of what is actually causing your symptoms. Which one are you presently treating, the symptoms, or the actual CAUSE?

(Endnotes)

[1] Rothmans R.H. and Slgoff. S: The effect of immobilization on the vascular bed of tendon. Surg. Gyenecol. Obstet. 124: 1064, 1967.

[2] Gelberman, R.H. m.d., Menon, J.M.D., Gonsalves, m.m.d., and Akeson, W.H.M.D., The effects of mobilization on the fascularization of Healing Flexar Tendons in Dogs. Clinical Orthopedics and Related Research, Number 153, Nov-Dec 1980

[3] Pekka Kannus, MD., PHD; Immobilization or Early Mobilization After an Acute Soft-Tissue Injury? The Physician And Sports Medicine; March 2000; Vol 26 No. 3, pp. 55-63

[4] John Nolte, The Human Brain, Mosby 1993, p. 139

[5] National Headache Foundation "Alternative Therapies and Headache Care"

[6] Corin M. Benneker, M.C., Paul Heini, M.D., Mauro Alini, PH. D., Suzanne E. Anderson, M.D., and Keita Its, MD., SC.D. 2004 Young Investigator Award Winner: VERTEBRAL ENDPLATE MARROW CONTACT CHANNEL OCCLUSIONS AND INTERVERTEBRAL DISC DEGENERATION. Spine Volume 30, Number 2. ppl 167-173. 2005

[7] Gianluca Cinotti, M.D., Carlo Della Rocco, M.D., Salvatore Romeo, M.D., Franco Vittur, M.D., Renato Toffani M.D., and Guido Trasimeni, M.D., DEGENERATIVE CHANGES OF PORCINE INTERVERTEBRAL DISC INDUCED BY VERTEBRAL END PLATE INJURIES. Spine Volume 30, Number 2, pp. 174-180 2005

[8] Markus Kroeber, M.D., Frank Unglaub, M.D., Thorsten Guegring, M.D., Andreas Nerlich, M.D., Tamer Hadi, B.A., Jeffrey Lotz, Ph. D., and Claus Carstens, M.D. EFFECTS OF CONTROLLED DYNAMIC DISC DISTRACTION ON DEGENERATED INTERVERTEBRAL DISCS. Spine, Volume 30. Number 2. pp. 181-187 2005

Chapter XIII

Prognosis
"Bout 10 Years"

Whiplash injuries occur daily. Can it be objectively determined if someone who is exposed to trauma, such as whiplash, has future symptoms as a direct result of their trauma?

Despite numerous studies, the prognoses of whiplash injuries remain controversial. The number of chronic symptoms varies according to the studies. Most studies indicate that a substantial proportion of patients still complain of neck pain and/or headache in the months or years after their acceleration-deceleration injury, which was usually caused by a rear-end collision. The factors predicting persistent chronic complaints are another source of debate. Litigation neurosis for financial gain has been proposed as the cause by a few authors. In contrast, other studies conclude that chronicity of symptoms is principally a consequence of initial severe and evolutive organic lesions. Studies on the prognosis of whiplash syndrome are numerous. Many of them are difficult to compare based on multiple methodologic differences such as selection criteria of patients, study designs, number of patients reviewed, length of follow-up, and therapy used. Moreover, a good number of these studies should be discarded because of their lack of meeting acceptable criteria of validity.[1.]

This is a great time to use Proverbs 4:7 and understand this chapter. Most research studies receive their results from subjective information, asking verbally or questionnaires taken by the patient. There are not objective exams, studies, such as EMG or video fluoroscopy to reveal any damage as a result of the accident.

Very commonly a patient will complain of headaches, neck and/or arm pain, and during the history state there was never any trauma to their neck. A lateral x-ray of the neck reveals a degenerated disc with local bone spur formation. [Figure 29]

During consultation, the patient will again not recall any previous neck trauma. When specifically asked about any, even minor car accidents, their number one response is "Bout 10 years ago I was in a little fender bender. I may have had a little pain and stiffness, but I didn't think I damaged my neck." It appears the accident damaged the intervertebral disc and ligaments, and this damaged area will reveal localized degeneration over time.

If prognosis of a whiplash victim is to be pondered, several questions must be considered.

1. Can the mechanism of injury (specifics of the actual accident) cause damage to the tissues involved?
2. What tissues were involved? (Ligaments, tendons, muscles, discs, facet joints, etc.)
3. Any objective findings substantiating the tissue damage? E.g. Ligament damage, seen on flexion/extension x-rays or video fluoroscopy revealing hyper mobility of the specific joint the damaged ligament is attempting to restrict.
4. Do the subjective complaints correlate with the objective findings? E.G. C5 facet damage should reveal symptoms relating to C5 dermatome.

Once you have the damaged tissue identified, the rest appears easy. All you have to do is know when that tissue heals back to normal and you have the prognosis. Or is the exact prognosis that simple?

The goal of this chapter is to get you to come to your own conclusion regarding the prognosis. Let us define prognosis and healing first.

Prognosis – A forecast of the probable course and/or outcome of a disease. (STEDMAN'S MEDICAL DICTIONARY)

Prognosis – Prediction OF the course and end of a disease, and the estimate of chance for recovery. (Taber's Cyclopedic Medical Dictionary)

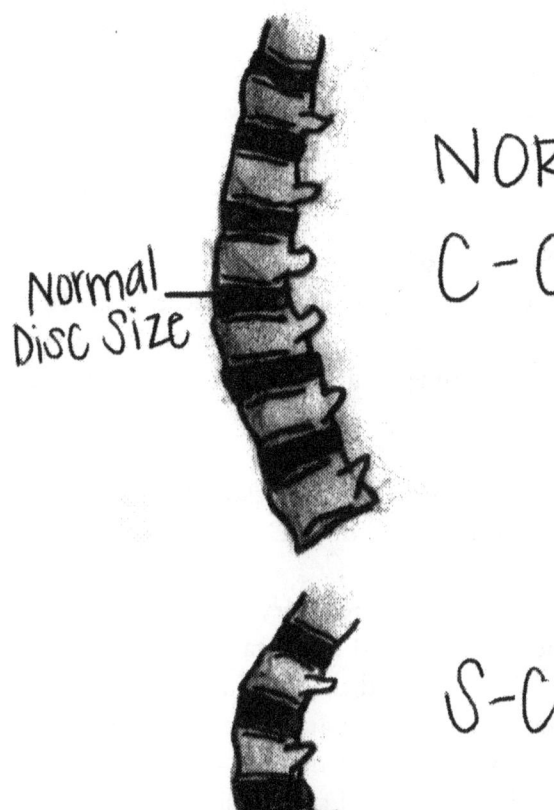

NORMAL
C-CURVE

Normal
Disc Size

S-CURVE

Bone
Spur

Degenerated
Disc

FIGURE 29

Healing – The restoration to a normal mental or physical condition, especially of an inflammation or a wound. Tissue healing usually occurs in predictable stages:

o Blood clot formation of a wound
o Inflammatory phase (during which plasma proteins enter the injured part).
o Cellular repair (with an influx of fibroblasts and mesenchymal cells).
o Regrowth of blood vessels (angiogenesis).
o Synthesis and revision of collagen complications: These may result from the formation of a scar that interferes with the functioning of a part and possible deformity. (Taber's Cyclopedic Medical Dictionary)

Healing – A process of cure. The restoration of integrity to injured tissue. (Dorland's Illustrated medical Dictionary)

If prognosis is estimated to the recovery or probable course, then when or how long does the damaged tissue take to heal? If healing is the restoration of integrity of injured tissue; when does that occur, and what about if someone is not hurting anymore? Does no pain mean they are healed? Let us look at one example.

Someone is involved in a rear end auto accident. Their ligaments surrounding C4/C5 (Anterior/posterior longitudinal ligaments) were stretched and slightly torn. Their symptoms correlated to C4/C5 dermatome levels. There is hyper mobility of C4/C5 during extension of their neck. Three months later, they are not in pain. There is no objective test, except for motion x-ray (video fluoroscopy) revealing continued hyper mobility of C4/C5 (posterior translation on extension). What is the prognosis?

If you are to guess at the prognosis, you first must look at the damaged tissue healing time. How long does it take a torn, normal type I triple Helix collagen fiber to return to normal integrity? That's the key question. How long, or does it ever return to normal? That's where the research should be targeted. If the ligament is not restored to normal, stretchy, and strong fibers, without scar tissue, the functional integrity of the joint is not restored. This is where the "Bout 10 years" comes in.

Let us take another example. During a typical rear-end collision, jamming of the facets and disc are noted in the studies. Let us say your patient reveals a C6 disc lesion. C6 nerve root pathology is present initially. After six months, this patient is not experiencing any pain or objective tests/signs. What is his prognosis? How long does it take a disc to heal, even though this person is symptom free?

For the record, I have never witnessed a disc lesion not degenerate and reveal years later a degenerated disc joint with bone spurs with the nerve root symptoms. I am not saying a damaged disc can not return to normal, I have just never witnessed a disc completely heal.

That is the needed research. Specific studies documenting specific lesions of tissue, following their course of recovery for years after the patient states they are symptom free.

When we get older, will we have neck pain and problems as a result of earlier trauma to our neck, or is the pain in my neck hereditary or my normal aging process? Let us look at an interesting study.

Objective – To determine the heritability of neck pain in persons 70 years of age and older.

Summary of Background Data – Previous studies have shown a moderate effect of genetic factors on back pain in the elderly. Genetic influence on neck pain in old age is unknown.

Results – A total of 2,108 twin individuals, including 1,054 complete twin pairs, answered the question related to neck pain at intake into the Longitudinal Study of Aging Danish Twins. Low and non-significant probandwise concordance rates, odds ratio, and tetrachoric correlations were found for both men and women in monozygotic and dizygotic twin pairs, indicating small or negligible genetic effects. Heritability estimates adjusted for age and significant environmental risk factors (rheumatoid arthritis, osteoarthritis, disc prolapse, and coronary heart disease) showed no significant additive genetic, dominant genetic, or common environmental effects.

Conclusion – Genetic factors do not play an important role in the liability to neck pain in persons 70 years of age or older. [2.]

The day after this chapter was written, a young lady stated she was moving out of the state. She wanted to take her x-rays with her. She had complaints of neck pain with headaches and her x-rays revealed a reversal of her cervical curve with extremely early signs of osteoarthritis in a couple of areas in her neck. When asked about past trauma to her neck, she stated "The only thing that happened was a little wreck about 10 years ago, but I was fine for years after that."

There's the key to this chapter. If research is performed by only asking subjective symptoms of the patient during the years of no symptoms, is this very accurate?!

Wouldn't it be great to see research include:

1. At the time of the accident – document subjective complaints with objective findings.
2. In about 10 years – document subjective complaints with objective findings.

Hopefully this research would include dynamic motion x-rays revealing any hyper mobility as a result of damaged ligaments. Of course, the best study would actually see the damaged ligament (not available at this time in the cervical spine). Maybe, just maybe, this research and other research would give us a hint of how long it takes for a ligament to heal (actually return to a normal collagen fiber), and if not heal 100%, reveal how close to normal this stretchy, tensile fiber gets.

Proverbs 4:7 – if you understood this book, the key to normal cervical biomechanics without any residual symptoms, is returning the damaged ligaments to its original dynamic normal cellular self, as well as the facet capsules and the intervertebral disc.

(Endnotes)

[1.] WHIPLASH INJURIES: Current Concepts in Prevention, Diagnosis, and Treatment of the Cervical Whiplash Syndrome, Michael Benorst: Dept. of Orthopaedic Surgery, Section of Rheumatology, Hospital Bequjon, University of Paris VII, Paris, France, Chapter II, p. 117.

[2.] Small Effect of Genetic Factors on Neck Pain in Old Age. A study of 2,108 Danish Twins 70 Years of Age and Older. Jan Hartvigsen, DC, PHD, Hans Christian Pederson, Msc, PHD, and Kaare Christensen, MD, PhD, Spine Volume 30. Number 2. Jan 15, 2005 pp.206-208

Chapter XIV

True Stories

True Story #1

I am a 54-year-old female. My name does not really matter, for I am sure there are many like me. Dealing with people who think I'm "FAKING" is really difficult. Thankfully, through working in a hardware store/lumber yard, I've met several people who know exactly what I'm going through.

At 33 years old, my second husband decided I was a good target to relieve his frustrations from life upon. The back of my neck took most of the abuse (I wore my hair long).

In 1993, I decided to leave under my own power instead of being carried out. I built a new life for myself. After almost four years, I finally got a property settlement, regular job, and thought I had it MADE. I only missed maybe ½ workday, one or two days a month because of neck pain. Yes, I had problems then, but for the most part, I could do anything I wanted to. I had even started back horseback riding. I loved to garden. I had grown nearly everything we ate when we were a family. I had milked a cow, made cheese; I was a HOME-STEADER. I was still clearing land and planning to add on to the house. I had a new man in my life. Things couldn't have looked much better. Then one day, after work, I was going to my friend's house. I was stopped at a yield sign and was hit from behind. There was no warning. The damage to my truck (S-10) was $1500.00.

The next day, when I went to get an accident report, I saw a sign that said there was a fee for a report in cash. I don't carry cash, so I went to the bank to cash a check. My hand wouldn't work. When I finally got my hand to work, I couldn't read my handwriting. I finally got through this, and got the wreck report to find no ticket had ever been issued.

I had no intention of anything other than getting on with my life, but found that my sense of balance and sight had changed. I found myself missing more and more work. I now have to take Ibuprofen for pain. I still have vision problems, balance problems, days when mentally concentrating just doesn't work. I also have excruciating neck pains at times as well as a total lack of energy (except at work, the "Public Face" takes over, but when I clock out, I'm exhausted). I now work six days a week, seven hours a day. I am so far behind at home you wouldn't believe. This is two and a half years later.

Driving, especially on rough roads, is very hard. God forbid speed bumps. I have had to just about quit gardening. Horse back riding, I realize is now a "pipe dream." Dealing with people who think I am faking is really difficult. Thankfully through working in a hardware store/lumber yard, I've met several people who know exactly what I'm going through. My usual problems are in my left upper back to mid back. It mostly aches (C4/5 dermatome). I have occasional headaches (sub-occipital).

FOR THE RECORD – This patient's head was slightly turned, looking for traffic, during the collision. Dynamic motion x-ray of the active range of motion of her cervical spine revealed moderate (significant) anterior translation of C4 or C5 during flexion (damage to longitudinal ligaments), foramenal encroachment (closing of vertebral foramina/where the spinal nerves exit) at C3/C4, C5/C6 on the left during extension. There was slight right lateral deviation of the Atlas on the Axis during right lateral flexion (damaged alar ligament).
If you would refer back to chapter VII, you should be able to match the damaged area with her symptoms using the affected nerves dermatomes. Example – sub-occipital Headaches – (damaged Alar ligament) – usual upper-mid back achiness (C4/C5 Anterior Translation).

Interesting note – x-rays revealed this lady had previously C5/C6 degenerated disc with osteo-arthritis (bone spurs) at that level. This arthritis restricted the movement at C5/C6. This restriction of movement at C5/C6 was prior to her auto-accident. The accident caused ligament damage to her cervical spine. Without question, most of the ligament damage was at C4/C5, the segments right above C5/C6.

TRUE STORY #2

In 1993, I injured my neck and right shoulder and back in a work accident. The injury to my neck has caused me the most difficulties and problems in the last 12 years than any other injuries.

I never had migraines before the accident. Now I get them quite frequently and they can be quite painful, virtually stopping me in my tracks. I have never liked heights, but I get dizzy and have vertigo on a two-step step stool. My balance is off. I can not walk a heel to toe straight line with my eyes closed, and sometimes not very well with them open either.

I used to wear contacts. One October I went in to have my prescription changed, picked up my contacts, and a week later I was back. They were wrong. I couldn't see to drive. I had a re-exam and changed the prescription. A week later the same thing happened. After four exams, I was blaming the doctor. Then I went to a different doctor, an eye specialist. My eyes were changing weekly, if not daily, due to the injury in my neck. For nearly a year I could not drive, and since then I have stuck with glasses.

If I read too much or do a lot of computer work, I can aggravate my neck. I will get pain in my last three fingers and sometimes my thumb. I've had pain radiate up through my jaw. The pain is always going down my back. The usual is a tight, achy pain in my upper back, between my shoulder blades. I regularly experience vision, balance, vertigo, headaches, back pain, arm and finger pain. All of this is from a neck injury. Who would have thought?

FOR THE RECORD – Dynamic motion x-ray of this patient's active cervical spine ranges of motion revealed posterior translation (hyper mobility/damage longitudinal ligaments) of C2 on C3, C3 on C4, and C4 on C5 during extension. There was a slight right lateral deviation (alar ligament damage) noted of the atlas on the axis during right cervical lateral flexion.

Chapter XV

Hope

Never, ever, ever give up Hope that you will find help for your symptoms. Keep searching for someone who can help you. The more I learn and know, the more I realize how much we don't understand about the human body. Every day research reveals more clues and answers to medical problems. Tomorrow may be the final solution to yours.

If you have a problem, hang in there. Help is around the corner. Never give up Hope.

In "THE SECOND NECK STEP," research data will be compiled documenting the loss of coordination/proprioception due to damaged neck mechanoreceptors. I do not believe that a highly trained, professional athlete just has a bad day and appears uncoordinated for one event. Could the answer be located in their mechano-receptors altering their proprioception?

www.ingramcontent.com/pod-product-compliance
Lightning Source LLC
Chambersburg PA
CBHW022009170526
45157CB00003B/1208